COMPREHENSIVE MEDICAL THESAURUS WITH CONCISE ETYMOLOGICAL ANALYSIS

W̶O̶R̶K̶B̶O̶O̶K̶ ̶F̶O̶R̶ C̶O̶N̶Q̶U̶E̶R̶I̶N̶G̶

```
REF. 610.14 O38c

Ohno, John M.

Comprehensive medical
   thesaurus with concise
```

DATE DUE

COMPREHENSIVE MEDICAL THESAURUS WITH CONCISE ETYMOLOGICAL ANALYSIS

WORKBOOK FOR CONQUERING MEDICAL ENGLISH

JOHN M. OHNO, Ph.D.

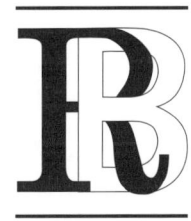

Rutledge Books, Inc. Danbury, CT

Copyright © 1999 by John M. Ohno

ALL RIGHTS RESERVED
Rutledge Books, Inc.
107 Mill Plain Road, Danbury, CT 06811
1-800-278-8533
www.rutledgebooks.com

Manufactured in the United States of America

Cataloging-in-Publication Data
Ohno, John M.
   Comprehensive medical thesaurus with concise etymological analysis

   ISBN: 1-58244-012-3

   1. Medicine -- Terminology.
2. Nomenclature.

610/ .1 /4

REF. 610.14 O38c

Ohno, John M.

Comprehensive medical
   thesaurus with concise

Contents

Preface vii

Introduction ix

Foreword xi

Part I: Classification of Thesaurus 1

    1. Introduction 3

    2. Identical Meaning with Different Combinations 6

    3. Examples of Mouth Inflammation Thesaurus 10

    4. Examples of Miscellaneous Medical Thesaurus 13

    5. Thesaurus of Medical Technology 15

    6. Examples of Thesaurus by Alphabetical Order 27

Part II: Analytical Study 135

    1. Analysis of Structure and Medical Modifier 137

    2. Etymology of Medical Compound Terminology 148

    3. Spelling Changes 159

    4. Grouping of Medical Prefixes by Meaning 164

    5. Prefixes by Alphabetical Order with Examples 173

    6. Suffixes by Alphbetical Order with Examples 239

    7. Linguistic Analysis of Medical Thesaurus 259

    8. Elemental Change of Location in Compound Words 270

    9. Examples of Analogy Between Prefixes and Suffixes 275

Part III: Quick Overview of Associated Medical Thesaurus 285

    1. Thesaurus Relating Psychoneurotic Disorders 287

2. Blood Pressure-related Thesaurus and Glossary 288

3. Respiratory-related Therapeutic Thesaurus 289

4. Dietary-related Thesaurus 289

5. Vitamin-related Thesaurus 291

6. Glossary Related to Natural Medicine 292

7. Examples of Pseudothesaurus 293

8. Thesaurus Relating Advanced Diagnostic Systems 294

9. Thesaurus Relating "Cata-" or "Meta-" 295

10. Thesaurus Relating Hormones 296

11. Thesaurus Relating Enzymes (or Protein Metabolism) 297

12. Thesaurus Relating the Thyroid Gland 299

13. Thesaurus Relating Blood Disorders 301

14. Thesaurus Relating Blood Vessels Disorder 303

15. Thesaurus Relating Dental and Oral Problems 305

16. Thesaurus Relating Neck, Shoulder and Spinal Disorders 310

17. Thesaurus Relating Major Skeletal Systems 318

18. Thesaurus Relating Cerebrovascular Disorders 320

Appendix **325**

1. Classification of Physicians 327

2. Classification of Medical Studies 329

3. Complex Thesaurus related to "Angioma" and Etymological
   Analysis 332

4. Examples of Similar Thesaurus and Pseudothesaurus 333

5. Thesaurus related to Heart Attack and Stroke 334

Index (for Part I) **336**

Preface

"The physician speaks a strange and often unintelligible dialect (which) creates a communication gap between the physician and patient that is acknowledged by neither."[1]

Dr. John Ohno is a man with extraordinary energies. His work on medical terminology has grown from years of experience with language, medicine, and consulting in translation in the worlds of both medicine and the law. He has broad interests, authored and edited a book on modern senryu[2]—in a collection of works by many authors—in which a number of the entries were written by Dr. Ohno himself. These writings offer only a small bit of insight into his broad range of interest and views of life.

Dr. Ohno's work on medical terminology, included in this extensive work, covers a broad range of problems in health care. He has organized materials by body systems, common disorders and on diagnostic as well as therapeutic terminology. He includes a linguistic digest to explain the origins of word roots used in medicine and has developed a section for acronyms and a medical thesaurus.

Dr. Ohno has undertaken a monumental task. Medical terminology is constantly changing. Biomedicine categorizes, labels, and subdivides at an extraordinarily rapid pace. As new terms and usage appear, other terms fall into disuse. Meanings and labels shift as medical sciences uncover and develop new technologies and approaches to human process. In addition, medicine itself has subdivided into a series of complex subcultures, termed subspecialties, each of which has special language, views, paradigms, and technologies. As a result, medicine has developed a language that is difficult enough for practitioners themselves.

For these reasons, medicine and medical practitioners could be said to have their own unique language, and the special terms that develop within language systems such as Japanese and English are often based on very different word roots and thereby construct realities differently. Equivalency is often hard or even impossible to achieve. Commonly used terms not only change their meaning, intent, and focus among practitioners, but they are frequently not 'common' in the language and day-to-day usage of patient populations.

As new technologies arise, or new diseases appear, new expectations and concerns appear in the clinical setting. Environmental contaminants, AIDS, cholesterol, and prostatic ultrasound-these are just a few of the issues of the past decade. They are popularized in the press, by TV, and on the radio. They are even incorporated into commercials, and later in questions and concerns that families and patients bring to clinics. Even well-defined terms, like allergy, develop a life of their own. Among English speakers, allergy has become part of the jargon individuals use to explain any number of personal and even social problems. Patients come to clinics using allergy to explain headaches, feeling tired, being depressed, losing weight, dysfunction at work, and so on.

Human concerns and fears are thus clothed in the garb and language of powerful systems-science and biomedicine-and underlying difficulties at home in relationships, and in life process masquerade in the guise of biologic dysfunction. This often serves to complicate communications in medical settings, because the meanings patients attach to illness episodes often grow from a focus that is not shared by the health practitioner they encounter.

Terminology almost inevitably requires explanation. Without this process, new terms (in any language) have limited meaning to the listener.[3] For this reason, single word or one-sentence equivalents serve primarily as labels, labels that may be devoid of real meaning when heard for the first time. Without explanation in language the patient can understand, meaning may be lost. Practitioners, patients, and bilingual workers in health care need to keep this in mind when they use special terms, reference a bilingual dictionary, or use a bilingual resource on terminology such as this one. Dr. Ohno's work offers us an excellent starting point for understanding terms and for learning about their origins as well as their interrelationships.

Robert W. Putsch, III, M.D.
Associate Clinical Professor of Medicine
University of Washington School of Medicine
Medical Director, Cross-cultural Health Care Project
Pacific Medical Center, Seattle, Washington

---

[1] Kimball, CP: Medicine and dialects. Ann Int Med 1971; 74:137-9.
[2] Ohno, Shuho: Modern Senryu in English. Seattle, Hokubei International, 1988. Shuho is his pen name.
[3] Werner O. Campbell DT: Translating, working through interpreters and the problem of decentering, in Naroll R, Cohen R (Eds): A Handbook of Cultural Anthropology. Irvington-on-Hudson, NY, Columbia University Press, 1973, pp. 130-171.

INTRODUCTION

In our rapidly changing world in which there is an increasing necessity for international collaboration, good communication in all disciplines has become extremely important. This is especially true in medicine and the health sciences in which there is constant development and refinement of current practices and investigative techniques. A good working knowledge of medical terminology provides a solid foundation for success and effective communication in medicine, the health sciences, and other related fields. Dr. John Ohno has devoted his life to the study of linguistics and medical terminology, and his efforts have resulted in the publishing of this excellent work.

Particularly, I would like to recommend this book as a textbook for students at medical and dental schools, pharmaceutical schools, nursing schools, and other health related fields, such as biochemistry, genetic science, rehabilitation, and public health (including epidemiology, environmental and occupational health, health services, international health, and biostatistics). It is essential for them to learn medical terminology as a basis for their own discipline. Furthermore, it will be extremely useful for Japanese students because Dr. Ohno has written the textbook with the intention that the book can also be used by many Japanese students who need to master medical terminology in English. His textbook will contribute greatly towards narrowing the gap in the understanding of medicine and the health sciences between health professionals, scientists, and students with different language backgrounds.

Tsukasa Namekata, Ph.D., Dr.H.Sc.
Director, Nikkei Disease Prevention Center
Clinical Associate Professor
School of Public Health and Community Medicine
University of Washington
Seattle, Washington, U.S.A.

Foreword

This book has been prepared to enrich your knowledge of medical thesaurus with etymological analysis to solve serious language barriers between lay people and medical professionals who use so many Greek and Latin terms. The knowledge derived from this book will help solve language barriers by avoiding confusions at the site.

Available medical terminology workbooks are mainly designed to train and test people in health care related occupations. But, the goal of this new book is to cover much broader areas such as lay people including ESL (English as Second Language) people, interpreters, and translators. America is very much a racially mixed society. Therefore, this workbook is very useful for ESL people as well as for everybody.

Citing some confusions among lay people regarding Greek and Latin thesaurus, most kidney specialists call themselves "nephrologist" based on the Greek word "nephros". But they also use Latin such as "renal biopsy", "renal calculus", "renal calyx" and "adrenal gland." All these words are related to the kidney. But, the adrenal gland is located above the kidney and belongs to the area of "endocrinologist".

Many thesaurus are generated endlessly in medical books and reports as medical science and technology develop. Therefore, this book is a *current overview of medical thesaurus and gives you a foundation for the future.*

John M. Ohno, Ph.D.

PART I

CLASSIFICATION OF THESAURUS

CHAPTER 1

INTRODUCTION

In 1852, Mr. Roget published a book titled *Thesaurus*. The first edition included synonyms, antonyms and other related words. Many people found it invaluable. Later, his son and dozens of editors revised the original edition. However, Roget's *Thesaurus* did not include medical terminology. Therefore, the author edited medical thesaurus for the first time.

If medical terms are combined with prefixes or suffixes, the medical thesaurus can be expanded extensively. However, the goal of this book is to publish a concise text and reference as a start.

Please note that some words are not up to date, because young and old physicians are using different terminology. The words are sometimes different depending on cultural background. Therefore, learning a variety of medical thesaurus is the key to solving language barriers in this racially mixed international society.

For example, "Muscular Dystrophy" is called "ALS" meaning "Amyotrophic Lateral Sclerosis" or many others such as "Progressive Spinal Muscular Atrophy," "Myotonic Myopathy," "Motor-Neuron Disease" (in Britain), "Aran-Duchenne Muscular Atrophy," "Lou Gehrigh's Disease."

<u>Linguistic Analysis of the above ALS Thesaurus</u>

Dystrophy: Defective nutrition syndrome (Dystonia: Muscular impairment)

Amyo: Muscular impairment

Trophy: Condition of nutriton (Atrophy or dystrophy means defective nutrition)

Lateral: means "side" (from Latin word: Latus)

Sclero: means "hard" (from Greek word: Scleros)

-sis: Suffix "sis" means "result" (Sclerosis: Hardened condition)

Myo-: prefix meaning muscular

-pathy: Suffix meaning illness (or suffering)

Related Thesaurus of Prefix and Synonym

Acronym: Head word. (Acro is a Greek word meaning extremity, and "nym" means "word."

Homonym: means "same word" (obsolete); Homo means "same."

Antecedent: Latin word meaning "in front of." (obsolete)

Pro: Greek word meaning also "in front of." (obsolete)

Pre: Latin word "prae" meaning "in front of." An example is "prefix."

Typical Examples of Medical Thesaurus Confusion

The thesaurus fibromyalgia and fibrositis are used differently by different groups in America. "Younger physicians, especially rheumatologists use the terms interchangeably. Old doctors tend to use fibrositis as a synonym for myofascial pain syndrome.

"We use the term fibromyalgia because it apparently is becoming more common and it avoids the suggestion of inflammation implied by the "itis" of fibrositis.

"Fibromyalgia has only recently gained recognition since 1990 as a distinct terminology. Rheumatoid arthritis has often been dismissed as an imaginary or psychiatric problem."[1]

"Fibrositis, a term coined by Dr. Gowers in 1904, has undergone a conceptual evolution over the last 88 years. For years, orthopedists, neurologists, neurosurgeons and physical medicine specialists termed fibromyalgia myofascial pain syndrome or musculoligamentous strain."[2]

---

1. Peng Thim Fan, M.D. and Margaret E. Blanton, M.D., The Journal of Musculoskeletal Medicine, April, 1992, p. 25.

2. Daniel J. Wallace, M.D., Op cit, Editorial Comment, p.3.

Table 1: List of Thesaurus Confusion

Terms	Spaces for adding own notes
fibromyositis	
fibromyalgia	
fibrositis	
myofascial pain syndrome	
musculoligamentous strain syndrome	
rheumatoid arthritis	

There are more examples related to "muscle inflammation" such as *"polymyositis"* (   ), *"dermatomyositis"* (   ), instead of using *"fibro"* but *"myo."* *"Poly"* came from the Greek word *"polys."*

The word Polymyalgia rheumatica" (   ) is an obsolete term, but *"rheumatoid arthritis"* (   ) is quite common among women. This is an inflammation of snyovial membrane (   ), so it is called *"synovitis"* (   ). Another confusion of thesaurus is the difference between *arthritis* and *rheumatism*. *Bursitis* (   ), *synovitis* (   ), and *tendinitis* (   ) are nonarticular rheumatism or called soft-tissue rheumatism. These are all localized inflammation caused by an accidental injury or overuse of a joint. On the other hand, arthritis is a chronic condition. Another confusing thesaurus is *"gouty arthritis."* This is not *"synovitis,"* but is called *"chemical crystal arthritis"* (   ).

CHAPTER 2

IDENTICAL MEANING WITH DIFFERENT COMBINATIONS

Thesaurus (synonym) is the group of words which *are related* to each other, but *not necessarily identical*. In this chapter some examples of *identical meaning* are edited. These examples with different prefixes or suffixes are also related to each other.

Example 1: Poor Digestion

    anapepsia (poor digestion)

    cacochylia (same)

    cacogastric (same)

    dyspepsia (same)

    oligopepsia (same)

Table 1: Linguistic Analysis of Example 1

Meaning of prefixes:	Meaning of suffixes:
ana (negative)	chylia (digestive juice)
caco (bad, ill)	gastric (stomach)
dys (bad)	pepsia (state of indigestion)
oligo (few, little)	peptic (digestion)

Example 2: Blindness

    ablepsy or ablepsia

    anopia or anopsia

    typhlosis

Table 2: Linguistic Analysis of Example 2

Meaning of prefixes:	Meaning of suffixes:
a (negative)	blepsia (sight)
an (negative)	blepsy (sight)
typhlo (blindness)	opia (visual condition)
	opsia (same)
	opsy (same)
	opy (same)
	sis (result, process)

Example 3: Anemia (See also page 29)

    <u>an</u>emia (lack of blood supply)

    <u>hypo</u>emia (same)

    <u>isch</u>emia (same)

    pancyto<u>penia</u> (deficient)

    thrombocyto<u>penia</u> (same)

Table 3: Linguistic Analysis of Example 3

    Prefixes

        an (deficiency)

        hypo (deficiency)

    Stems

        isch (poor blood supply)

        pancyto (cellular elements)

        thrombocyto (platelet)

    Suffixes

        emia (blood condition)

        hemia (blood condition)

        penia (deficiency)

Example 4: Neuroblastoma

Glioblastoma is also called spongioblastoma.

    glioblastoma

    spongioblastoma

Table 4: Analysis of Example 4

Prefixes:	Suffix:
blasto (embryonic)	ma (tumor)
neuro (nerve)	
glio (gluey)	
spongio (resilient)	

Example 5: Oophoron and Ovary

a) Identical Meaning

ovaritis and oophoritis

ovarian cyst and oophorocystosis

Stems	Suffixes	Meanings
ovary	itis	inflammation
oophoron	cystosis	cyst formation

Note: Ovarian or ovary means egg, "ovum" in Latin. Oophoron also means "ovary," but the origin is Greek.

b) Thesaurus with different suffixes

Thesaurus	Suffixes	Meanings
ovariocentesis	centesis	perforation or puncture
ovariotomy	tomy	surgical incision
ovariectomy	ectomy	surgical removal
oophorectomy	ectomy	surgical removal
oophorosalpingectomy	ectomy	surgical removal
oophorocystosis	cystosis	cyst formation
salpingioma	ma	tumor
salpingitis	itis	inflammation
salpingocyesis	cyesis	pregnancy
ovariocyesis	cyesis	pregnancy
salpingopexia	pexia	fixation
salpingostomy	stomy	surgical opening
ovariostomy	stomy	surgical opening

Note: Salpinx means "tube" in Greek. "Salping" in this case means "ovarian tube."

CHAPTER 3

Examples of Mouth Inflammation Thesaurus

(Suffixes: -itis, -asis, -osis) and ulcer or sore, etc.

1) Aphthous stomatitis

   itis (means inflammation in Greek.)

   aptha (means eruption in Greek.)

   stoma (means mouth in Greek.)

2) Aphthous ulcer (also called "Mouth Ulcer")

   ulcus (inflammatory crater in Latin.)

3) Canker sore (also called "Mouth Ulcer")

4) Candidiasis or Candidosis

   Candidus or Candida is a name of fungus in Latin.

   osis (pathological condition in Greek)

   Cause: Candida fungus

   Symptoms:

   inflammation

   bleeding

   pruritus

   white exudate

5) Oral thrush (One of candidiasis)

   Cause: Candida fungus

   Symptom: white exudate

6) Oral Herpes (also called "Herpes Simplex")

   Cause: Virus infection

   Symptoms: blisters on lips

   painful ulcers

7) Cold Sores

   Herpes Simplex on the lip

8) Oral Cancer

   Symptom: neoplasm on the lip or in the mouth.

Throat Inflammation Thesaurus

1) <u>Aden</u>algia or <u>Adeno</u>dynia

   Aden or adeno means "gland" in Greek.

   Adenocele

   Adenofibroma

   Adenoid

   Adenolipoma

   Adenolymphoma

   Adenoma or Adenosarcoma

   Adenomycosis

2) Tonsillitis

3) Adenopharyngitis or Pharyngitis

<u>Tooth-Related Inflammation Thesaurus</u> (see also pg. 306)

1) Gumboil (Painful swelling called "fistula")

2) Gingivitis (Inflammation of the gum)

3) Alveolitis

4) Pulpitis

CHAPTER 4

EXAMPLES OF MISCELLANEOUS MEDICAL THESAURUS

Related Words	Medical Thesaurus	Individual Language Notes
longitudinal section divide right and left	sagittal	
divide front and back	anterior (front) posterior (back)	
cross-sectional above below	transversal superior inferior	
to the center from the center near to the center far from the center	afferent efferent proximal distal distad	
toward middle away from the middle	medial lateral	
prefix meaning side	latero lateroabdominal lateroflexion	

Related Words	Medical Thesaurus	Individual Language Notes
toward the tail toward the head	caudad cephalad	
prefix meaning head	cephal cephalo	
move a limb away from the body	abduction abductor	
front toward front back toward back back side	anterior ventral posterior dorsal, dorso notal	
right, heart	dextro, dextrocardia, dextrum, cordextrum	
left, heart	levo, levocardia	
Prefix meaning middle *	meso, mesocardium	

* see also page 85

CHAPTER 5

THESAURUS OF MEDICAL TECHNOLOGY

Some thesaurus are found in diagnostic, therapeutic, and surgical technologies. As mentioned in previous chapters, these are either identical or related.

Group A: Diagnostic Thesaurus

Example 1: Doppler Scanning

The change in the observed frequency of sound as a result of movement is called the Doppler effect, which is used in medical ultrasound scanning.

Thesaurus:

Echocardiography

Ultrasound Scanning

Example 2: Telepathology

This group of diagnostic techniques by use of television monitor or telemetry monitor is called "Telepathology."

Thesaurus:

Digital Fluoroscopy (   ), Digital Angiography (   )

Thermography

Example 3: Computer Tomography (CT) or Computer Axial Tomography (CAT)

This is a cross-sectional imaging using a ray detector and computer.

Thesaurus:

Magnetic Resonance Imaging (MRI)

Open-sided MRI

> This is based on Nuclear Magnetic Resonance (NMR) which is the reaction of the body's hydrogen in a powerful magnetic field. No X-ray is involved in this technique.

Positron Emission Tomography (PET) (also called PET scanning)

> Positrons are introduced into the body and PET scanning produces three-dimensional images. Radioisotopes are injected into the blood.

Single-Photon Emission Computed Tomography (SPECT)

> Gamma-ray detectors rotate around the patient while scanning.

Nuclear particle "proton" is used as a powerful source for "MRI-Tomography", called "NMR".

Example 4: Diagnostic X-ray, Scanning X-ray

- Angiocardiogram
- Chest X-ray
- Cholangiopancreatography
- Mammography
- Venogram (or Phlebogram)

Example 5: Electrograph

- AEG: Atrial Electrogram
- ECG: Electrocardiogram
- EDG: Electrodynograph (for walking, jogging, climbing)
- EEG: Electroencephalograph (for brain waves)
- EHD: Electrohemodynamics (for vascular system)
- EKG: Electrocardiogram

VEG: Ventricular Electrogram

Example 6: Auscultation

    Auscultatory Percussion

    Direct Percussion

    Finger Percussion or use of Plexor (　　　)

    Fetoscope

    Stenoscope

    Phonocardiogram (　　　) by use of electroacoustic device

Group B: Scopy by Use of Diagnostic Scopes

    Arthroscopy (　　　) by use of an endoscope (　　　)

    Bronchoscopy (　　　) by use of fiber-optic device

Types of Scopes:

    Abdominoscope

    Anoscope

    Colonoscope

    Colposcope

    Culdoscope (　　　): for examination of Cul-de-sac (　　　)

    Cystoscope

    Duodenoscope

    Endoscope

    Endoscopic Retrograde Cholangiopancreatography

Fiberscope

Gastrocamera

Hysteroscope

Laparoscope

Sigmoidoscope

Group C: Catheterization

Cardiac Catheterization or Heart Catheter

Hepatic Vein Catheterization

Laryngeal Catheterization

Female Urethra Catheterization

Foley Catheter (Double-lumen cuffed catheter)

Male Urethra Catheterization

CAT-CAM: Contoured Adducted Trochanteric Controlled Alignment Method

Various Catheters:

Angiocatheter

Atherectomy with a rotating scraper

Balloon Catheter for atherectomy

Catheter with a guide wire

Cutaneous Catheter

Foley Catheter (Dr. Foley's rubber catheter with a balloon tip)

Single-Hole Catheter or Multiple-Hole Catheter

Swan-Granz Catheter with a tiny balloon tip for open-heart surgery.

Group D: Therapeutic Dialysis, Diffraction Process

Continuous Ambulatory Peritoneal Dialysis

Fistula Hemodialysis

Immunoadsorption Dialysis by use of Prosorba

Group E: Radiation Therapy

Example 1: Laser

Laser: Amplification of Stimulated Emission or Radiation

There are Argon-laser, CO2 laser, YAG laser

YAG (Neodymium-Ytrium-Aluminum-Garnet)

Applications:

CO_2 laser for treatment of bronchial disorder

Cancer treatment

Cutaneous treatment

Retinosis treatment

Stone removal without surgery

Example 2: Radiation Therapy or Actinotherapy

Types:

Implant

Interstitial Radiation

Intracavitary Radiation

External Radiation by use of X-ray or Gamma ray

Group F: Surgical Thesaurus

Example 1: Tomy (Incision) Operation

    Cecotomy

    Costotomy

    Craniotomy

    Enterotomy

    Episiotomy

    Fasciotomy

    Herniotomy

    Hysterotomy

    Ilectomy

    Keratotomy

    Laparotomy

    Lithotomy (Lithotripsy)

    Myotomy

    Pericardiotomy

    Phlebotomy or Varicotomy

    Thoracotomy

    Tracheotomy

    Typhlotomy

Vagotomy

Example 2: Ectomy (Excision) or Resection (also called Segmentectomy)

    Adenectomy

    Appendectomy

    Bowel Resection

    Carcinectomy

    Cholecystectomy

    Colectomy

    Cystectomy

    Embolectomy

    Endarterectomy

    Enterectomy

    Hemorrhoidectomy

    Hydrocelectomy

    Hysterectomy

        Abnominal, Fibroid, Vaginal Hysterectomy

    Laryngectomy

    Liver Resection

    Lobectomy

    Mastectomy

    Nasalpolypectomy

    Nephrectomy

Parotidectomy

Pneumonectomy

Proctectomy

Prostatectomy

Stomach Resection

Tonsillectomy

Typhlectomy

Vasectomy

Example 3: Ostomy (Stoma) Operation

Anastomosis

Cecostomy

Cecostigmoidostomy

Cholecystostomy

Cystostomy

Enteroanastomosis

Enterostomy

Gastrostomy

Ileostomy

Thoracostomy

Tracheostomy

Example 4: Fistura Operation

Most of these operations are abnormal passage operations except Fistula Hemodialysis.

    Branchial Fistura

    Cervical Fistura

Example 5: Centesis Operation or Paracentesis

Thesaurus: Perforation, Pricking, Puncture

    Abdominal Centesis

    Amniocentesis

    Pericardiocentesis

    Thoracocentesis

    Venepuncture

    Venesection

Example 6: Cerclage sutura, or Surgical Stitches

This operation is to close wounds or incisions.

Thesaurus:

    Buried Sutura

    Cervical Suturing also called Cerclage

Interrupted Sutures:

Each stitch is tied at the side.

Mattress Sutures:

For deeper wounds, the needle is passed through the wound twice.

Cerclage: Hooping of fractured bone

Stapling:

    An automatic stapling device is used. This operation is very efficient. Staples are easily removed later.

Sutura Dentata:

    An immovable fibrous join for connecting bones of the skull.

Sutura Limbosa:

    An immovable fibrous join for parietal and temporal bones.

Sutura Serrata:

    An immovable fibrous join similar to Sutura Dentata, or Sutura Limbosa.

Group G: Absorptiometry Thesaurus:

This is a group of Bone Mass Density tests.

    1. Single Photon Absorptiometry Test
    This test counts the absorption of photons passed through bones such as the forearm bone and heel.

    2. Dual Photon Absorptiometry Test
    This test can separate mineral mass from soft tissue mass, used for hip and spine.

    3. Quantitative Computed Tomography
    This CAT scan is for spine.

    4. Dual Energy Absorptiometry
    This is similar to DPA, but it uses X-ray radiation.

Group H: Liposuction Thesaurus

    1. Cosmetic Liposuction
    A cosmetic surgeon removes fat from the body.

2. Liposuction with soft-tissue surgery
Performed by a dermatology surgeon.

3. Ultrasonic Liposuction
An ultrasonic probe inserted through a tube.

4. Tumescent Technique
Local anesthesia combined with sedation.

5. Wet Technique
General anesthesia or heavy sedation.

Group I: Genetic Engineering Thesaurus

    1. Artificial fertilization or gestation, genesis

    2. DNA suction

    3. Cell division or cloning

    4. Meiosis, Mitosis (see chapter 6, Section M)

    5. Nuclear division

    6. Implantation

Group J: Heart-Related Miscellaneous Technique

    1. Angioplasty and Bypass surgery
    Balloon angioplasty
    Enlargement of a narrowed heart valve

    Laser angioplasty
    Ultrasound to break up blood clots

    2. Defibrillator
    Electro-tipped catheter

    Implantable cardioverter defibrillator

    3. Pericardiocentesis

Removal of excess fluid from the sac surrounding the heart.

Group D: Therapeutic Dialysis (see also pg. 19)

1. Dialysis Thesaurus

"-lysis" means a technique of loosening substances from a solution such as contaminated blood by the difference in the rate of diffusion. It is called "dialyzer." The technique is called "hemodialysis".

a) Kidney dialysis

b) Peritoneal dialysis

2. Types of dialysis technique

a) Artery-vein fistula

b) Femoral vein hemodialysis

c) Subclavian hemodialysis

3. Related disorder

a) Dialysis dementia

b) Dialysis disequilibrium syndrome

Note: As medical technology develops day by day, some of the above operations in this chapter are becoming obsolete, and new technology is quickly taking over to replace them.

Please also note that this chapter is a very condensed summary for this concise text/workbook.

CHAPTER 6

Examples of Thesaurus by Alphabetical Order

Section A

Related Words	Thesaurus	Examples	Own Notes
abdomen	belly celia celio flank laparo peritoneal venter (Latin)	abdominal pain bellyache celiac block celioma flankache laparotomy peritoneum peritonitis ventral	
aberrant	chromatic aberrant mental aberrant		
ablate	abortion remove	removable	
abnormal	aberration anorma	abnormality chromosome aberration anormal	
above	superior	aboveboard superior maxillitis	
accumulate	accumulation agglutination ascites calcus edema	anthracosis asbestosis agglutinin ascites praecox ascites adiposus chylous ascites renal calcus cardiac edema purulent edema	

27

Related Words	Thesaurus	Examples	Own Notes
achylia	achlorhydria achylosis hypoacidity		
acyesis	infertility sterility		
aden	adeno lymph node	adenitis adenocarcinoma adenocele adenoid lymphadenitis	
addisonism	adrenal crisis	Addison's disease	
adrenal	adrenalin adreno epinephrine	adrenal cortex adrenal hormone adrenocortical	
aerophagia	aerophagy belch crepitus eructate flatulence flatus	belching crepitation eructation	
agenesia	agenesis cacoepy (obsolete)		
aging	agnosia Alzheimer's disease apraxia atrophy catabiosis decrepit dementia Parkinson's disease senile	agnosis amnesia decrepitude senile dementia continuous tremor senility	
akathisia	ADD restlessness	attention deficit disorder	

Related Words	Thesaurus	Examples	Own Notes
aliment	alimentation nutrient	alimentary nutrition nutritious	
allergy	allergic anaphylactic atopic hypersensitive	allergic asthma allergic rhinitis anaphylaxis atopic asthma atopic eczema atopic dermatitis hypersensitivity	
albumin	protein	aluminoid protein metabolism proteinuria	
amnesia	dementia		
anabolic	anabolism anabolite steroid	buildup metabolism muscle buildup	
anal atresia	anal stenosis anal stricture		
analgesia	acetaminophen lytic cocktail nerve block painkiller	analgesic cocktail anasthetic	
anaphylaxis	allergy hypersensitivity	anaphylaxia	
anastomosis		arteriovenous fistula	
androgen	anabolic hormone testosterone	anabolic steroid	
anemia	aplasia	anemia aplastic anemia hemolytic anemia megaloblastic	

Related Words	Thesaurus	Examples	Own Notes
anemia (cont'd)	bone marrow aplasia chlorosis hypoemia iron deficiency anemia ischemia pancytopenia thrombocytopenia pernicious anemia	aplastic anemia hypovolemia Raynaud's ischemia	
anesthesia	 analgesia	anesthesiologist local anesthesia regional anesthesia topical anesthesia analgesics	
aneurysm	artery aneurysm berry aneurysm brain aneurysm varicose aneurysm	aortic aneurysm cerebral aneurysm	
ankle	tarsus	ankle edema tarsalgia	
ankyle	amphiarthrosis ankyla arthrosis	cartilaginous joint ankylosis arthrodesis	
anodyne	analgesia antalgic antispasmin sedative	 sedative hypnotic	
anoxia	hypoxemia	anemia anoxia	
anticoagulant	blood thinner	heparin	
antidiuretic	A.D.H. hormone vasopressin	A.D.H.	

Related Words	Thesaurus	Examples	Own Notes
antidote	antitoxin antivenin		
apex	apic apicectomy apical tip	apex beat apex cardiogram apex cordis apex pulmonis apical pulse root amputation apical curettage tiptoe	
aphonia	dysphonia dysphemia	dysphasia	
aphrasia	aphasia		
apheresis	pheresis	leukapheresis plasmapheresis	
aphrodisia	aphrodisiac libido	bisexual libido libido sexualis	
appendix	cecum	appendicitis cecitis typhlitis	
arm	axillary brachial	armpit axillary lymph node brachial artery	
aroma	fragrance perfume		
artery	aorta aortic aortic body aortic aortitis	aortarctia (obsolete) aortectasia (obsolete) aortic aneurysm aortic arch syndrome carotid body aortic stenosis aortitis syndrome	

Comprehensive Medical Thesaurus

Related Words	Thesaurus	Examples	Own Notes
artery (cont'd)	aorto	aortoclasia aortomalacia aortostenosis	
	aortopulmonary arterial	fenestration of — arterial insufficiency of extremities	
	arterial	arterial PH	
	arterial	arterial pressure	
	arterio	arteriography arteriomalacia arteriosclerosis	
	arteriovenous	arteriovenous angioma of the brain arteriovenous fistula arteriovenous shunt	
	arteriole	arteriola	
	arteritis	endarteritis endaortitis periarteritis rheumatoid arteritis temporal arteritis	
	artery	artery forceps	
arthritis		osteoarthritis rheumatoid arthritis	
	arthrocele arthrochondritis arthrodynia	arthrocentesis bursitis rotator cuff tears tendinitis	
	osteomalacia		
articular		articular cartilage articular fracture	
	articulatio	articulatio cubiti (elbow joint) articulatio genus (knee joint)	

Related Words	Thesaurus	Examples	Own Notes
articular (cont'd)	(gliding joint) articulation artus cartilage junction	articulatio plana joint joint cartilage graft cartilage joint junctura synovialis (synovial joint)	
aspiration	suction	aspirating abscess	
asthenia	adynamic debility myasthenia		
asthma	 dyspnea wheezing	bronchial asthma paroxysmal dyspnea	
atele	atelia (obsolete) atelo atelectasis ateliotic dystrophy	ateleiosis (obsolete) atelocardia atelocephalous postoperative atelectasis ateliotic dwarf dystrophia	
athiaminosis	beriberi kakke disease		
atony	atonia atonic diskinesia flaccid impotence	atonia constipation colon stasis fecalith inactive colon lazy colon atonic impotence flaccid bladder	
atopic	allergic atopic	allergic dermatitis atopic asthma	

COMPREHENSIVE MEDICAL THESAURUS

Related Words	Thesaurus	Examples	Own Notes
atresia	atreto closure coarctation constriction occlusion stenosis	uterine atresia atretolemia atretometria traumatic occlusion aortic stenosis stenothorax	
atrophy	atrophic cachexia dystrophy pernicious	atrophic fracture cachexy muscular dystrophy pernicious anemia	

attack	apoplexy
	arrest
	attack
	epilepsy
	infarction
	paroxysmal
	
	seizure
	stroke
		apoplectic stroke
		respiratory arrest
		heart attack
		epileptic attack
		cerebral infarction
		paroxysmal
		  dyspnea
		motor seizure
		cerebral
		  hemorrhage
		heat stroke	

auscultation	stenoscope		
autopsy	necropsy thanatopsy	thanatology	
avulsion	tearing		
axillary	armpits	axilla axillary node	
azoospermia	infertility oligospermia spermacrasia sterility	insufficient sperm poor sperm	

Section B

Related Words	Thesaurus	Examples	Own Notes
back	dorsal dorsi dorso notal stooping	backache dorsalgia dorsiflexion dorsodynia notalgia kyphosis	
bacteria	bacterial bacteremia botulism mycobacteria Neisseria salmonella	bacterial aneurysm mycotic aneurysm food poisoning mycobacteriosis Neisseria meningitis salmonellosis	
bag	alveoli alveolus aneurysm appendix bursa cecum cyst diverticulum follicle gallbladder ovary pouch sac saccular saccule air saccules scrotum urocyst vesicle vesicular	alveolar air dental alveolus arterial aneurysm appendectomy bursitis cystectomy diverticular folliculitis ovarian cyst blind pouch gestational sac saccular aneurysm sacculus scrotal cancer urocystis seminal vesicle vesicular emphysema	
bald	alopecia atrichia atrichosis		

Related Words	Thesaurus	Examples	Own Notes
bane	bane germ intoxicate poison toxicity venom virus	baneful poisonous toxin envenom	
bath	balneology balneal	balneotherapy	
belching	eructation	(see aerophagia)	
below	inferior lower	inferiority complex lower abdomen	
bile	bile biliary bilirubin chole gall icterus jaundice	bile duct biliary cirrhosis bilious bilirubinuria cholelith gallstone	
biliary calculi	cholelith cystic duct stone		
birthmark	nevus	naevus	
bladder	cyst vesicle	bladder stone cystolith vesical calculus	
bleed	bleeder emptysis entorrhagia epistaxis hematemesis hemorrhage hemorrhoid	hemophilia hemoptysis cerebral hemorrhage gastric hemorrhage	

Related Words	Thesaurus	Examples	Own Notes
bleed (cont'd)	menorrhagia menses nosebleed	menstruation	
blind	ablepsia anopia typhlosis	ablepsy anopsia	
blind gut	cecitus cecum typhlectomy	cecitis cecotomy typhlitis	
bloat	filling swelling		
block	nerve block	celiac block	
boil	carbuncle folliculitis furuncle	furunclosis	
bottom	fundus	fundus hemorrhage uterous fundus	
brain	cerebellum cerebro cerebrum dextrocerebral diencephalon encephalo interbrain thalamus	brain concussion cerebrosclerosis cerebral concussion encephaloma thalamic syndrome hypothalamus	
break	crack disconnect fissure fracture split	splitter	
breast	mammary	breast-feeding mammary cancer	

Related Words	Thesaurus	Examples	Own Notes
breast (cont'd)	mammilla mast	mammitis mastadenitis mastalgia mastatrophia mastectomy mastodynia	

breathing	aspiration
	breathing
	eupnea
	exhalation
	inhalation
	respiration
		neonatal breathing
		
		artificial respiration
		abdominal
		  respiration
		internal
		  respiration*
		cellular respiration*
		neonatal
		  respiration	

breech	buttocks gluteal	gluteal tuberosity	
brittle	brittle bone fragile frail	bone fracture osteoporosis fragility frailty splinter	
bruise	black eye contusion		
bubble	follicle globule vacuole	globulus	

*Note that internal or cellular respiration is quite different from normal respiration. The oxygen exchange takes place between the blood and body tissue calls. The oxygen given to the blood is used for metabolic activities as an energy source.

Related Words	Thesaurus	Examples	Own Notes
bucca	cheek	buccal	
bug	insect pest vermin	insecticide pestiferous verminosis	
bulimia	gross overeating	bulimia	
buttocks	gluteal	gluteus	
bypass	bypass graft shunt sidetrack	artery bypass	

Section C

Related Words	Thesaurus	Examples	Own Notes
caked breast		lactation mastitis	
calcification	calcitonin calcium calculus		
calculus	calculus cytolith litho	calcinosis renal calculus cytolithiasis lithocytotomy	
calyx	pyelo	caliectasis pyelocystitis pyelogram	
callosity	bony deposit callus	callous osteophytes callosity	
calmant	calmative sedative	sedation	
calvities	alopecia baldness calvous		
calyx	calix	renal calix	
calx	calcemia	hypercalcemia Ca rich blood	
canal	channel duct	alimentary canal channel ulcer duct ectasia	
cancellous	porous spongy	porous bone spongy structure	
cancer		benign cancer malignant cancer	

Related Words	Thesaurus	Examples	Own Notes
cancer (cont'd)	cancerous carcinogen carcinoma celioncus epithelioma leukemia lymphoma myeloma oncocyte oncogene oncology oncoma (obsolete) oncosis (obsolete) sarcoma squamous tumor	canceration Hodgkin's disease	
candidiasis	systemic candidiasis thrush		
canker sore	aphthous canker	aphthous stomatitis aphthous ulcer	
cardiac arrest	asystole	cardiac standstill	
caries	necrotic tooth decay	necrosis	
carpal	wrist	carpus	
cartilage	chondral periosteum	chondritis chondroarthritis protective membrane	
castrate	emasculate oophorectomy sterilization tubal ligation vasectomy	emasculation	

Related Words	Thesaurus	Examples	Own Notes
cataplexy	narcolepsy	sleep attack	
catatonia	catatonic stupor dystonia	catatonic schizophrenia	
cathartic	abreaction catharsis cathartics cleansing coprogogue lavage laxative purgation	psychocatharsis anocathartic bowel evacuation peritoneal lavage purging	
cavity	cavernous cavitas cavity follicle sinus	 nasal cavity thoracic cavity hair follicle sinusitis	
cecitis	cecal cecitis cecoptosis cecosigmoidostomy cecostomy cecotomy typhlitis typhlostenosis typhlotomy	cecum typhlostomy typhlenteritis	
cell	cellular clone cyto	 cellulitis polyclone	
cell division	cloning cytokine meiosis mitosis	divided duplication cytokinesis meiotic division	
centesis		abdominocentesis	

Related Words	Thesaurus	Examples	Own Notes
centesis (cont'd)	perforation puncture	thoracocentesis	
chancre	chancre chancroid chlamydia gonorrhea herpes genitalis syphilis		
change	alteration mutation transform	alterative gene mutation	
cheek	bucca	buccinator	
chest	pectoral stetho thora thoracic thoraco thorax	chest tube pectoralis stethoscope thoracostomy thoracic aorta thoracoabdominal	
chest muscle	pectoralis thoracic muscle		
chiasma	chiasm crossover		
chiro	chiroplasty chiropodist chiropractic	podiatrist chiropractor	
chloroma	granulocytic sarcoma green cancer		
chlorosis	anemia	iron deficiency anemia	

Related Words	Thesaurus	Examples	Own Notes
choking	asphyxia suffocation		
cholangioma	bile duct cancer		
cholecyst	gallbladder	cholecystitis	
cholesterol	adipose adipositas atheroma cholesterin fat lipo lipoprotein	adiposis adipositas hepatica atheromatosis lipids lipoma high-density lipo low-density lipo	
chorea		Huntington's disease	
cilium	eyelash		
clavicles	collarbones		
cloning	anaphase cell division clone genetic engineering mitosis nuclear division	DNA clone genesis	
closing	atelectasis atresia atreto clot embolic embolism infarction infarction stenosis thrombus	urethral atresia atretometria blood clot embolic stroke pulmonary embolism ileus infarction anemic infarction cardiac stenosis thrombosis	

Related Words	Thesaurus	Examples	Own Notes
clot	embolism stuffing	blood clot infarction plug	
cold	febris fever influenza pyrexia sinusitis	feverish flu	
color blindness	achroma chromic	achroma vision chromatelopsia chromic myopia	
colp	colpalgia colpocele colpodynia vagina	colpitis colpocytis colpolypus colpopathy vaginitis	
coma	comatose lethargic	diabetic coma lethargy	
comedo	acne family		
compulsion	obsession		
computed tomography	CAT scan	computed axial tomography	
conceptus	embryo fetus		
condom	prophylactic rubber		
condyloma	wart	venereal wart	
conjunctival test	allergy test		
conjunctivitis	pink eyes red eyes	eczematous- conjunctivitis	

Related Words	Thesaurus	Examples	Own Notes
connective tissue	cartilage	fibrous connective tissue	
contagious	contagion bacterium communicable epidemic infectious mycobacteria pestiferous salmonella virus	contact dermatitis bacteremia sex-related diseases influenza AIDS mycobacteriosis pathogenic salmonellosis viral infection	
corn	callus keratosis	callosity	
cornea	kera	keratitis keratoma	
cornual pregnancy	ectopic pregnancy interstitial pregnancy		
cortisol	adrenal hormone corticosteroid corticotropin hydrocortisol steroid	adrenocorticotropic hormone	
cortisone	glucocorticoid glycogenesis		
costal	ribs steno thoracic	stenocostal thoracic cavity	
Cowper's gland	Bartholin's gland bulbocavernosus muscles bulbourethral gland Cowper's gland	vaginal lubrication vaginal sphincter seminal secretion urethral sphincter (male)	

Related Words	Thesaurus	Examples	Own Notes
Cowper's gland (cont'd)	Skene's gland (female) vestibular gland	vaginal lubrication	
crepitus	belch flatulence	crepitation	
CRF	ACTH corticotropin release factor	release by the pituitary release by the hypothalamus	
Crohn's disease	ileitis	enteritis	
crypt	follicle	sebaceous crypt hair follicle	
cut off	cripple disfigure mutilate separate	mutilation separation	
cut open	cesarean dissect ectomy fenestrate incision lacerate tomic tomy window centesis	cesarian section dissection hysterectomy fenestration cut into an organ laceration dermatomic somatomic thoracotoy open window surgically ovariocentesis	
cyesis	gestation gravida pregnancy		
cyst	bladder cyst pouch	cystalgia cystectomy	

Comprehensive Medical Thesaurus

Related Words	Thesaurus	Examples	Own Notes
cystic fibroma	fibrous tumor myxofibroma myxomatosis	myxoma fibrosum myxomatous fibrosum	
cystic fibrosis	defective gene exocrine gland disorder chronic lung infection obstructive airway disease fibrocystic pancreas mucoviscidosis rejection of nutrient	inherited disease	
cystic neuroma	false neuroma neoplasm of the nerve tissue		
cystoma	neoplasm neoplasia sarcoma tumor	neoplastic osteosarcoma	

SECTION D

Related Words	Thesaurus	Examples	Own Notes
dacry	tear duct	dacryadenitis dacrygelosis	
decay	decomposition deterioration caries disintegration putrefaction rotten spoil	dental caries putrefy	
degenerate	atrophy decrement degenerative deteriorate diminish emaciation enervate exhaust prostrate	atrophic fracture decline uterine contraction osteoarthritis malnutrition enervation exhaustion prostration	
delivery	labor partus	parturition	
dementia	Alzheimer's anomia decrepit Down's syndrome senile		
dental	dental caries gingivitis orthodontia prosthodontics	dental decay periodontitis malocclusion denture	
dextro	right	dextrocardia	
dialysis	blood dialysis	hemodialysis	

49

Comprehensive Medical Thesaurus

Related Words	Thesaurus	Examples	Own Notes
dialysis (cont'd)	dialyzer	peritoneal dialysis	
diaphragm	partition phren	diaphragmatic hernia phrenospasm	
diarrhea	celiorrhea lientery		
diathesis	familial tendency	inherited susceptibility bleeding diathesis hemophilia	
dichotomy	division separation	two equal parts pairs	
dicumarol	anticoagulant		
digest	absorption assimilate metabolism	intestinal absorption metabolize	
digital	digital images	digital angiography	
digitalis	cardiotonic	digitalis therapy	
dilate	distend ectasia enlarge insufflation swollen	dilator distention ectasis	
disinfect	clean sanitize sterilize		
disperse	administer dispersing	drug administration dispersing agent	
dissect	anatomize	anatomization	

Related Words	Thesaurus	Examples	Own Notes
dissect (cont'd)	decompose dissect	decomposition dissector	
diuretics	chlorothiazide Diuril	thiazide diuretics urine excretion loop diuretics osmotic diuretics	
dizziness	giddy vertigo	giddiness cerebral vertigo	
dope	heroin marijuana morphine narcotic		
Doppler imaging	ultrasonography	echocardiography	
dormant	inactive incubation latent	incubation period latent cancer	
dorso	back dorsal	dorsodynia lumbodorsal	
dosage	fatal dosage megadose	booster dosage lethal dosage drug megadosing	
drivel	drool saliva	drooling	
dry	siccant siccus xero	dryer siccative siccus rhinitis xerostomia	
duct	canal channel duct	canalis pyloric canal channel ulcer (peptic ulcer) cystic duct	

Related Words	Thesaurus	Examples	Own Notes
duct (cont'd)	lumen pipe tube	duct ectasia vas deferens (pl) lumina, lumens pipette fallopian tube	
dysentery	amebiasis Shiga's bacillus shigellosis	amebic dysentery bacillary dysentery Shigella	
dyslexia	alexia alexis	inability to read no speech, no word	
dyspepsia	anapepsia cacochylia oligopepsia	cacogastric	
dysphagia see page 321	achalasia aphagia cockscrew esophagus dysphagia	sphincter trouble difficult swallow difficult swallow difficult swallow	
dysphonia	aphasia dysarthria dysphasia dysphrasia	diffective speech poor articulated speech poor speech poor speech	
dyspnea	apnea gasp panting stridor tachypnea wheezing	apneustic breathing rapid, shallow breathing stridulent	
dysthymia	bipolar depression chronic depression delusion manic depression	major depression hopelessness depressive psychosis	

Section E

Related Words	Thesaurus	Examples	Own Notes
ear	auris otis oto	auriscope otitis otoscope	
earlobe	auricle	auricula	
eczema	eczematous tinea	atopic dermatitis eczema herpeticum tinea capitis	
eliminate	dialysis discharge evacuate excision excrete extract secrete	dialysis fluid evacuation lithotomy excretory extractor secreted fluid	
elytro-	elytrocele vagino-	elytrostenosis vaginitis	
embryo	fetus embryoectomy	abortion feticide	
emission	eject ejaculation emesis emission excretion exudate secretion vomit	ejector ejaculatory duct nocturnal emission excreta exudation	
endarteritis	endaortitis		
endocardial	endocardium	endocarditis	

Related Words	Thesaurus	Examples	Own Notes
endometrial	endometrium endometriosis	endometrial cancer endometritis	
endoscope	arthroscope bronchoscope colonoscope cystoscope gastroscope laparoscope		
endotracheal tube		balloon catheter cardiac catheter drain catheter	
enema	cathartic	rectum injection	
enteral	intestinal visceral	enteritis intestinal ischemia visceral pain	
entering	afferent	afferent vessels	
enterocele	diverticulosis hernia	diverticulitis abdominal hernia	
entero-	colon entero intestinal	colonic fistula enteritis intestinal dyspepsia	
epidemic	communicable contagious infectious pandemic pestiferous	communicable disease	
epinephrine	adrenalin epinephrine	vasoconstrictor adrenal hormone	
episio	perineal perineum vaginal	episiotomy perinectomy vaginitis	

Related Words	Thesaurus	Examples	Own Notes
erythema	erythroderma roseola rubeola	erythematous	
esophagus	gullet lemo	esophagus cancer lemostenosis	
estrogen	follicle stimulating hormone lutenizing hormone progesterone		
etiology	pathology	etiologic pathogenesis	
eucrasia	euesthesia eugenics euphoria	euthenics	
euthanasia	assisted suicide mercy killing		
excite	excitation rejuvenation stimulation		
excrete	excrement expectorate fecal mucus saliva sputum stool	expectoration feces excretion of mucus lienteric stool	
exocrine gland	apocrine gland eccrine gland sebaceous gland sudoriferrous gland sweat gland	sebaceous crypt sebaceous cyst	

Related Words	Thesaurus	Examples	Own Notes
expansion	dilation ectasia insufflation stretcher	dilator gastrectasia stretch receptor	
exudate	exudation oozing pus		
eye	ocular ophthalmia orbital	ocular myopathy ophthalmitis orbital pseudotumor	

Section F

Related Words	Thesaurus	Examples	Own Notes
face lift	plastic surgery rhytidoplasty	rhytidectomy	
faint	delirium stun swoon (obsolete) syncope unconscious		
fascia	epimysium epithelium fascia perimysium	fibrous sheath covering tissue fasciectomy	
fat	adipo lipa lipid lipo lipoid lipocele obese sebaceous steato	adipose lipacidemia lipase lipoatrophy lipoiduria adipocele lipoma lipopexia obesity sebaceous layer steatoma	
fatigue	exhaust prostration		
feces	decrement excrete stool	steatorrhea	
feeble	debility infirmity weakness weariness	debilitation	
female	feminine	feminist	

Related Words	Thesaurus	Examples	Own Notes
female (cont'd)	lesbian muliebrity	female homosexual muliebral	
fertile	fecundate fecundity	fecundation	

fertilization	insemination
	oogamy
	pregnancy
		artificial
		  insemination
		oogenesis
		See "gravid"
		  Section "g"	

fetus	embryo fetalis		
fever	febricity febrile pyrexia yellow fever	febris Q fever	
fiber	cellulose fiber fibril fibrin filament	dietary fiber fiberscope fibrillation fibrinogen filamentation	
fissure	cleft crevice fissura fissure fistula laceration rima splint split tear	cleft lip fissurapudendum fistulectomy torn wound rimaglottis splinter	
flank	flank side	flank pain	
flesh	flesh meat		

Related Words	Thesaurus	Examples	Own Notes
flexible	bendable flexion flexure yield	joint flexion dorsal flexure	
fluid	liquid	amniotic fluid liquefaction	
flutter	fluctuation pulsation vibration		
follicle	folliculus vesicula	ovarian follicle folliculoma vesicule	
food poisoning	bacterial poisoning botulism clostridium endotoxin bacteria E. coli (0-157) egg poisoning endotoxin poison mushroom poison salmonellosis sausage poison shellfish poison	bacillus, etc. clostridium botulism Escherichia coli Salmonella phalloidine poison	
frailty	adynamia asthenia atrophy debility frailty		
front	anterior facial	facial plain	
fundus (Latin)	basal base bottom fundus	basal metabolism fundus uteri	
fungus	fungate	fungal infection	

Comprehensive Medical Thesaurus

Related Words	Thesaurus	Examples	Own Notes
fungus (cont'd)	mycosis	fungicide mycobacteriosis	
funic	funic funiculus	funicular umbilical cord	

Section G

Related Words	Thesaurus	Examples	Own Notes
galactic	galactocele lacteal	lacteal gland	
gallstone	biliary calculus cholelith	biliary stone	
gamete	meiosis	sexual cell sexual cell division	
gamo	conjugate gamogenesis marriage sexual union	conjugation reproduction	
ganglion	nerve cell neuroploca		
gastric	acid reflux gastrectasia gastrostomy heartburn peptic ulcer stomach ulcer	gastroreflux	
gastroenteric	gastrointestinal	gastroenteritis	
gay	homosexual lesbian	female homosexual	
gaze	stare	gaze palsy fixed stare	
genitals	genitalia pubic	genital reflex pubic region	
germ	bacteria microbe plague virus	*See Section "b"* microorganism white plague viral hepatitis	

Comprehensive Medical Thesaurus

Related Words	Thesaurus	Examples	Own Notes
gestation	cyesis fertile gravid pregnancy	cyetic *See Section "f"*	
gigantism	acromegaly gigantism huge	adenohypophysis gigantoblast growth hormone	
gland	glandula glandular	adrenal gland areolar gland ciliary gland thymus gland glandular carcinoma	
glans		glans clitoris glans penis	
glucosuria	glycosuria		
gluteal	buttocks gluteous	gluteal muscles	
glycogen	glucagon glucose glycerin glyco saccharogen	glucagon hormone glucose tolerance test glyceryl alcohol glycosuria saccharin	

goiter	Hashimoto's
	  disease
	
	sturuma
	thyroiditis
	thyrotropin
		sturuma
		  lyphmatosa
		thyroidectomy
		thyroid stimulating
		  hormone	

gout	gouty pseudogout tophus	gouty arthritis chondrocalcinosis	

Related Words	Thesaurus	Examples	Own Notes
graft	grafting transplant	artery graft isograft skin graft	
gravid	gestation gravid pregnant	primigravida gravidness	
groin	inguinal iliac region	inguinal hernia inguinodynia	

Section H

Related Words	Thesaurus	Examples	Own Notes
hair loss	alopecia	alopecia areata	
halitosis	breath smell malodorous breath		
hallucination	deception delusion fantasy hallucinosis illusion imagination	alcoholic hallucinosis	
hangover	nausea		
Hansen's disease	leprosy		
hay fever	allergic anaphylaxia	allergic rhinitis	
headache	cephalalgia cerebral concussion migraine headache		
hearing	acoustic auditory otalgia otitic oto	acoustic trauma auditory nerve otitis otocleisis otopyorrhea otoscopy	
heart	cardia cor coronary heart heartburn	cardiac arrest cor dextrum coronary disease heart attack congestive heart failure gastro-acid indigestion	

Related Words	Thesaurus	Examples	Own Notes
heart (cont'd)	myocardial	myocardial infarction	
helper cell	lymphocyte suppressor T cell		
hem	blood (haima) blood clotting hemato hematology	erythrocyte hem analysis hemagglutination hematochezia hematocrit	
hematoma	blood blister	blood clots	
hematoplastic	hematopoiesis	erythropoiesis	
hemicrania	migraine headache		
hemiplegia	hemiparaplegia hemiparesthesia hemiplegia	hemiparesis cerebral hemiplegia facial hemiplegia spastic hemiplegia	
hemolysis	aplastic anemia hemolysis	hemolysin	
hemostasis	blood clotting embolism hemostasis hemostatic thrombosis thrombus vasoconstriction	mechanical hemostatic	
hemotroph	embryotroph hemotroph	histotroph hemotrophic nutrition	
heparin	blood thinner heparin	anticoagulant heparin rebound	
hepatalgia	cirrhotic liver		

Related Words	Thesaurus	Examples	Own Notes
hepatalgia (cont'd)	hepatic coma hepatitis hepatocirrhosis		
hepatitis	acute hepatitis A chronic hepatitis hepatitis A hepatitis B hepatitis C hepatitis D	viral hepatitis cirrhosis, fibrosis viral infection serum infection (HIV) serum infection, serious new development	
hereditary	atopic congenital genetic hereditary inherited	atopic asthma atopic dermatitis congenital amputation genetic disorder hereditary ataxia inherited disorder	
hernia	diverticulum femorocele hiatus protrusion	diverticulosis hiatus hernia	
herpes	eczema herpeticum herpes labialis	Kaposi's varicelliform eruption herpes simplex	
herpes zoster	 varicella shingles	herpes zoster virus chicken pox	
heterogeneous	allograft conglomerate diverse hetero- heteroeroticism	cross-fertilization heteroplasm heterosexual alloeroticism	
hiatus	 opening membrane	hiatus hernia gastroesophageal reflux	

Related Words	Thesaurus	Examples	Own Notes
hiccup	hiccough singultus		
hirsutism	hirsute hypertrichosis shag	shaggy	
HIV	retrovirus		

hives	prurigo
	prutitus
	shingles
	urticaria
	wheal
		pururigo simplex
		pururitus
		  universalis
		herpes shingles
		  virus
		urticaria
		  pigmentosa	

hole	calix crypt fistura foramen meatus	renal calix anal fistura bone foramen auditory meatus	
homeo	same homeotypic	homeopathy homeostasis homeotypical	
homogeny	homogeneous homogenetic homograft	homogenesis	

hormone
(see pgs. 296, 297)
	anabolic steroid
	corticosteroid
	estrogen
	follicle
	  stimulation-
	  hormone
	lutenizing hormone
	oxytocin
	progesterone
	testosterone
	thymosin
		FSH	

Related Words	Thesaurus	Examples	Own Notes
hormone (cont'd)	thyroid hormone		
hormone therapy		endocrine therapy	
hump	stoop spinal curvature	humpback stooping kyphosis lordosis	
hybrid	combination genotype hybrid crossbreed mongrel	hybrid computer mongrel animal	
hyperplasia	enlargement hypertrophy megalo megaly	adaptive hypertrophy megaloblast megaloureter gastromegaly	
hypophysis	pituitary		
hypothyroidism		Grave's disease	
hypoxemia	anoxemia anoxia hypoxemia	acute hypothemia apnea coma cyanosis stupor	

Section I

Related Words	Thesaurus	Examples	Own Notes

iatrogenic	nosocomial
	
	nosopoietic
		iatrogenic disease
		nosocomial
		  infection
		nosopoietic
		  infection	

icterus	jaundice		
ileitis		Crohn's disease ileotomy	
ileostomy	colostomy enterostomy ostomy	surgical opening	
imagination	deception delusion fantasy illusion		
immune	homeostasis immunization interferon pasteurize vaccination	immune response immune therapy inhibiting protein pasteurization	
impediment	obstruction		
incontinence		bowel incontinence reflex incontinence stress incontinence urge incontinence urinary incontinence	
infarction	cerebral infarction myocardial infarction	stroke heart attack	

Related Words	Thesaurus	Examples	Own Notes
infarction (cont'd)	embolism thrombosis vasoconstriction		
inflammation	aphthous stomatitis alveolitis candidiasis gingivitis oral herpes colitis ileitis pharyngitis	aphthous ulcer gumboil	
infectious	contagious communicable epidemic infectious prosodemic	 influenza AIDS	
infusion	infiltrate injection insufflation	infusion pump blow a gas into	
insanity	lunacy psychosis	psychotic disorder	
inside	centrocyte centripetal endocardinal endoscope entoderm implant inter intra	centesis centrum ascending current cardiac pacemaker endoprosthesis gastroscope endoderm implantation internist intracutaneously	
insomnia	agrypnea anhypnea awake-deep sleep vigilance	insomniac vigilant	

Related Words	Thesaurus	Examples	Own Notes
instability	lability unstable	emotional lability labile	
integument	cutaneous epidermis skin	cutaneous anaphylaxis cuticle skin graft	
intention	autonomic intention	autonomic nervous intention tremor	
intercourse	coitus conjugation copulation pareunia zygogenesis zygosis	union of gametes sexual reproduction	
intersexual	bisexual hermaphroditism promiscuous	bisexual libido hermaphrodism	
intertrigo	erythematous skin irritation	red skin infection	
intestinal	intestine intestinal lipodystrophy	digestive tract intestinal infarction intestinal dystrophy	

intravenous	intravenous bolus
	intravenous
	
	venipuncture
	
	venotomy
		intravenous push
		intravenous
		  feeding
		intravenous
		  infusion	

introduction	infusion injection incision instillation insufflation	intravenous injection phlebotomy	

Related Words	Thesaurus	Examples	Own Notes
inverse	invert reverse	inverse anaphylaxis reversible reaction	
ipsilateral	homolateral	same side	
ischemia	aplasia anemia chlorosis hypoemia iron deficiency ischemia pancytopenia pernicious anemia thrombocytopenia	aplasic anemia hemolytic anemia young women's anemia hypovolemia chlorosis ischemic lumbago thrombocytopathy	
itchy	pruriginous prurigo mitis prurigo agria prurigo ferox pruritus	pururitic prurigo simplex severe prurigo pururitus cutaneous pururitus localis	

Section J

Related Words	Thesaurus	Examples	Own Notes
jargon	aphasia jargon aphasia	gibberish aphasia mixed aphasia jargonize	
jaundice	icterus	infectious icterus	
jaw	chin jaw mandible	jaw bone mandibular	
joint	anastomosis articulatio cubiti articulatio plana artus (obsolete) joint junction synovial joint	elbow joint gliding joint joint cartilaginous joint junctura synovitis	
juice	succus	succorrhea	
jugular	jugulum larynx neck pharynx throat	jugular vein	
juxta	beside juxta juxtaposition near	juxtangina juxtamural juxtaspinal	

Section K

Related Words	Thesaurus	Examples	Own Notes
kakke	athiaminosis beriberi	thiamine deficiency	
kakosmia	cacosmia kakidrosis osmidrosis		
kera	callus callosity gout horn kera osteophytes processus	callous urate crystals horniness keratitis keratoiditis keratoma	
kidney	nephr renal	nephritis renal calculus	
kleptomania	cleptomania stealing habit		
knee	genu genu varum kneecap knock-knee	articulatio genu bowleg patella genu valgum	
kyphosis	kyphoscoliosis	spinal curvature	
kysthitis	colpitis vaginitis		

Section L

Related Words	Thesaurus	Examples	Own Notes
labia	folds labia labio lips nympha nympha pudendum	labia majora labia minora labiodental nymphitis nymphomania external genitalia	
lacrimal	tear	lacrimal duct tear duct	
lactase		lactase deficiency alactasia	
lactation	breast-feeding galact lacteal mammary gland	galactorrhea lacteal gland breast	
lactose	galactose glucose lactin		
lalio	laliatry lalio lalopathy stuttering	laliophobia lalopathology speech dysfunction	
lamina	lamella laminar layer membrane stratum basale stratum corneum stratum lucidum stratum spinosum	membrana basal layer horny layer clear cell layer prickle cell layer	
lavage	peritoneal dialysis	peritoneal lavage	

Related Words	Thesaurus	Examples	Own Notes
lavage (cont'd)	dialysis	gastric lavage	
learning disability	attention deficit disorder dysgraphia dyslexia		
lethargy	hypnosis lethargic narcolepsy	hypnotics drowsiness	
lentigo	freckle macula	tan macule juvenile lentigo maculation	
lentivirus	retrovirus	AIDS virus	
lesbian	gay	female homosexual	
lesion	boil lesion rash skin injury wound	furuncle irritative lesion local skin injury primary skin injury	
leucocyte	leukocyte leukocytopenia leukocytosis leukophoresis leukopoiesis	white blood cell leukopenia basophilia eosinophilia neutrophilia leukocytogenesis	
leukopathia	leukocytoma leukoderma leukoma leukoplakia leukosis leukotoxin leukorrhea	 white skin white patches vaginal discharge	
leukemia	leukopenia	leucocytopenia	

Related Words	Thesaurus	Examples	Own Notes
leukemia (cont'd)	leucocythemia leukemia cutis	leucocytosis lymphoderma perniciosa	
leukotomy	lobotomy	brain neurosurgery	
libido	 erotomania libidinous masochism onanism	bisexual libido eroticism lustful algolagnia sadism, sadomasochism masturbation	
lingo	jargon lingua lingual lingual term	jargon aphasia tongue lingual papilla terminology	
lining	membrane pleura synovial tendon sheath sheath	mucus membrane serous membrane synovial membrane nervous sheath	
linitis	 leather-bottle stomach	linitis plastica	
lipa	adipocele adipose fat lipid	lipocele adipose tumor lipoma fatty acid cholesterol	
lipo	lipoatrophy lipodystrophy lipoma lipomyoma lipopenia lipoprotein liposuction sebacious	 lipomatosis liposarcoma sebacious gland	

COMPREHENSIVE MEDICAL THESAURUS

Related Words	Thesaurus	Examples	Own Notes
lipo (cont'd)	tallow		
lithiasis	biliary stone calculus calcus cholelithiasis lithiasis lithogenesis lithotomy microlithiasis	biliary calculus calculus anuria urinary calcus gallbladder calculus renal calculus calculus excision cholelithotomy alveolar microlithiasis	
livedo	mottle lupus livedo	cutis marmorata livedo reticularis netlike mottle	
liver	hepatic hepato hepato	alcoholic cirrhosis hepatic cirrhosis hepatitis portal cirrhosis hepatocholangitis hepatogastritis	
lobe	portion of any organ lobectomy lobotomy lobular	anterior lobe (pituitary) frontal lobe (head) intermedius lobe (pituitary) medium lobe (lung) occipital lobe (head) posterior lobe (pituitary) chest surgery leukotomy lobular carcinoma	
lochia	lochial discharge	postpartum discharge	

Related Words	Thesaurus	Examples	Own Notes
lochia (cont'd)	lochio	lochiometritis lochiorrhagia	
loin	flank loin lumbar lumbar waist	lumbago lumbar puncture lumbar vertebra	
lues	syphilis	syphilitic aortitis	

lung	
	pneumo
	
	pneumato
	pulmonary
		lung cancer
		pneumococcus
		pneumonia
		pneumatocele
		pulmonary
		  carcinoma
		pulmonary edema
		pulmonary
		  embolism
		pulmonary stenosis	

lupus	discoid lupus
	  erythematosus
	  (DLE)
	lupus
	  erythematosus
	
	lupus vulgaris
	sarcoidosis
		
		systemic lupus
		  erythematosus
		  (SLE)
		tuberculosis (skin)
		lupus pernio	

lymph	lymphadenitis lymphadenopathy lymphangitis lymphatic lymphocytes Two forms of lymphocytes	 lymphatic gland lymphatic leukemia lymphocytopenia lymphocytosis lymphocytotoxin B cells T cells	

Comprehensive Medical Thesaurus

Related Words	Thesaurus	Examples	Own Notes
LSD	lysergic acid		
lysis	dissolution lysin lyso	dialysis lysotype	
lyssa	lyssin lyssoid lyssophobia	dog bite poison crazy dog disorder rabies vaccine	

SECTION M

Abbreviation	Meaning depending on the case	Own Notes
MA	mental age, menstrural age, etc.	
MAB	monoclonal antibody	
MABP	mean arterial blood pressure	
MAC	maximum allowable concentration minimum alveolar concentration	
MAC Awake	recovery time from anesthesia	
MAP	mean arterial pressure	
MAST	mastectomy	
MBC	maximum breathing capacity maximum bladder capacity	
MBL	menstrual blood loss	

Related Words	Thesaurus	Examples	Own Notes
macerate	soaking	maceration macerator	
machismo	abusive macho virile	dominating trait masculinity virility	
macilent	emaciate	emaciation	
macrencephaly	macrocephaly macroencephaly macrocephalia	macroencephalic	
macrocytosis	anisocytosis microcytosis poikilocytosis	anisopoikilocytosis	

Related Words	Thesaurus	Examples	Own Notes
macro	macrocyte macrocytic macromolecule	macrocytic anemia	
macrophage	phagocyte phagocytosis	fixed phagocyte free phagocyte engulf microorganism	
male	androcyte androgen homosexual masculine virile virilism	 gay virility adrenal virilism	
mal	malabsorption malocclusion malignant malnutrition malodorous malpractice virulent	weight loss malignant tumor malignant state	
mania	crazy maniac manic hysteric	andromania pedophilia sex maniac kleptomanic manic-depressive hysteric mania	

marrow	bone marrow
	myeloblast
	
	myelocyte
	
	myelocytic
		
		myeloblastic
		  leukemia
		immature white
		  blood cell
		myelocytic leukemia	

masochism	algolagnia nymphomania sadism sadomasochism	sexual perversion	

Related Words	Thesaurus	Examples	Own Notes
mastalgia	breast pain mastitis	mastalgic pain acute mastitis chronic mastitis	
masturbation	onanism self-stimulation		
measles	roseola rubella	German measles rubeola	
meatus	opening passage tunnel	acoustic meatus nasomeatus nasopharyngeal meatus	
meiosis	anaphase interphase metaphase telophase	meiotic division nuclear division final stage of division	
melancholia	depression	agitated depression	
membrane	diaphragm interseptum lining membrana membrane meninges peritoneum pleura	endorcardium membrane pleura lining membrana tympani membrane diffusion mucous membrane meningitis abdominal serous membrane serous membrane of the lung	

Related Words	Thesaurus	Examples	Own Notes
memory loss	amnesia anomia aphasia dementia	Alzheimer's disease	
meno (disorders)	amenorrhea menometrorrhagia menorrhagia menostasia menoxenia oligomenorrhea	menolipsis abnormal bleeding hypermenorrhea menostasis abnormal menses hypomenses	
meno (aging)	menopause	cessation of menses	
menses	catamenia menorrhea menstrual menstruation	normal discharge menstrual cycle menstrual period	
mental displeasure	anhedonia dysthymia	melancholia	
mentality	mental capacity mental deficiency	mental retardation Down's syndrome	
metastasis	growth metastasis metastatic transmission	growth of cancer metastatic calcination	
metra	metro metrocele uterine	metralgia metrocarcinoma uteralgia	
middle	inter mean medial median medium mesa mesen	interseptum mean arterial pressure mesaraic mesencephalon	

Related Words	Thesaurus	Examples	Own Notes
middle (cont'd)	mesenterial mesial meso metaphase middle	mesenteritis mesoderm middle ear	
migration	metastasis MIF (migration inhibitory factor) migration transmission transposable	metastatic cancer migratory pain transmigration transposon	
mitosis	clone indirect division meiosis metaphase mitosis	 sex cell division homeotypic mitosis multipolar mitosis	
morbid	morbidity patho- morbus pathosis	morbid anatomy illness pathogen pathogenesis diseased pathology	
motor seizure	epilepsy focal seizure convulsion		
mucosa	mucous membrane		
mucus	mucin mucinous mucoid mucoserous mucosa mucous myxo-	colloid carcinoma mucinous carcinoma mucinoid mucocutaneous mucous membrane myxoadenoma myxofibroma	

Related Words	Thesaurus	Examples	Own Notes
mucus (cont'd)	myxoid myxoma	mucoid or mucinoid myxofibroma	
multigravida	multipara		
multiple gene	polygene		
multiple myeloma	plasma cell myeloma		
multiple personality	schizophrenia split personality		
murmur	 arrhythmia fibrillation flutter	aortic murmur cardiac murmur thoracic murmur arterial fibrillation cardiac fibrillation	
muscle	muscular muscular tumor musculo musculus my- myo- achalasia pectoralis seizure	muscular dystrophy muscular sarcoidosis myoma musculoskeletal system musculus bucinator myalgia myotrophy myotonia pectoralis major pectoralis minor convulsive seizure	
myoatrophy	amyotrophy dystrophy myotonic	 myotonic myopathy	

Section N

Related Words	Thesaurus	Examples	Own Notes
nanism	dwarfism nanosomia nanus		
narcotic	anesthetic anodyne narcoplepsy narcosis narcotic opiate palliate sedative stupor	anodynia sleep paralysis insensibility narcotic analgesics opium narcotic drug palliative treatment anergic stupor delusion stupor epileptic stupor	
nausea	seasick vomit	vomiting vomitory	
navel	umbilical		
nebulizer	atomizer nebulization sprayer		
neck	cervical cervix neck pylorus	cervix uteri neck dissection pyloricstenosis	
necroscopy	autopsy		
necrosis	dead tissue gangrene	necrotomy dry gangrene	
nephron	kidney nephralgia	kidney dialysis nephritis	

Comprehensive Medical Thesaurus

Related Words	Thesaurus	Examples	Own Notes
nephron (cont'd)	nephropathy ren	renal failure renal biopsy	
nerve	nerve block neuroglia neuralgia neuron	anesthesia neurology neuronitis axoneuron	
nervous breakdown	depression hypochondria melancholia stupor	manic depression hypochondriasis bipolar disorder	
nervus	nervus facialis nervus olfactorius nervus opticus	facial nerve olfactory nerve optic nerve	
neuropath	neurasthenia neurosis nervous exhaustion	fatigue neurosis	
neurosis	insanity mental disorder neurotic disorder obsession paranoia psychoneurosis psychosis	mania paranoid disorder major mental disorder	

nitroglycerin	nitrospan
	
	nitrostat
		angina pectoris
		  relief
		coronary
		  vasodilation	

nocturnal	night nocturnal nyctal	night blindness nocturnal emission nocturia nyctalopia nycturia	
nosebleed	epistaxis rhinorrhagia		

Related Words	Thesaurus	Examples	Own Notes
noso	disease nosocomial nosocomial infection path	nosology hospital nosophobia pathology	
nostalgia	homesick nostalgic nostomania		
Novocain	local anesthesia		
noxa	noxious poison toxin toxo	poisonous toxocariasis	
nucleus	base center core kernel		
nuisance	annoyance		
numbness	analgesia palsy paralysis plegia stupefaction	cerebral palsy spastic paralysis cycloplegia	
nutrient	alimentation nourishing threpology	nutriment nourishment sitology	
nympha	labia minora nympha	nymphitis nymphomania nymphotomy	

Section O

Related Words	Thesaurus	Examples	Own Notes

obese	adipose
	corpulent
	obesity
	
	ponderous
		adipositas
		corpulence
		hyperplastic
		  obesity
		hypertrophic
		  obesity
		overweight	

obligate	compulsive obligate	compulsive neurosis obligate aerobe obligate anaerobe obligate parasite	

obsession	allurement
	attraction
	captivation
	compulsion
	crash
	enchantment
	fascinate
	frenzy
	infatuation
	mania
	obsess
		compulsive
		  neurosis
		
		infatuate
		
		obsessive
		  personality	

obstetrics	gynecology obstetrics	gynecologist obstetrician obstetric anesthesia	
obstetrix	midwife	certified midwife	

obstipation	constipation	atonia constipation
		colonic
		  constipation
		perceived
		  constipation
		rectal constipation	

Related Words	Thesaurus	Examples	Own Notes
obstruction	angina block choking clogging clumping coarctation constricting embolism emphysema ileus impediment narrowing plug stasis stenosis stroke suffocation	angina pectoris nerve block respiratory choking artery clogging artery coarctation pulmonary embolism adynamic ileus vessel narrowing nasal stuffiness circulation stasis	
occipital	hemicrania occipital headache		
occlusion	closing obturation occlusion	obturator malocclusion traumatic occlusion	
occult	dormant insidious latent occult	insidious AIDS latent carcinoma occult blood occult fracture	
oculo-	ocular optic orbital retinal	ocular myopathy optic nerve orbital aperture retinitis	
odonto-	dental odont odontitis	dentist odontalgia toothache	
oil gland	sebaceous sebaceous gland	sebaceous crypt	

Related Words	Thesaurus	Examples	Own Notes
oil gland (cont'd)	sebum		
olfaction	osphresis osphresio- sense of smell	anophresia odors ospheric	
oligemia	hypovolemia hypoxemia		
oligo-	oligogenesis oligopepsia oligospermia oliguria	birth control indigestion poor digestion azoospermia	
omo-	shoulder omodynia	shoulder ache	
omphalo-	omphalocele navel umbilicus	congenital hernia omphaloectomy umbilectomy	
onanism	masturbation	masochism	
oneiro	delusion dream oneirodynia oneirogmus	delusions of grandeur oneirology nightmare nocturnal fantasy sleep terror nocturnal emission	
onychi	 onychialgia nail unguis	onichia	
oogamy	fertilization heterogamy oosperm		
oophoron	 ovarian	oophoritis ovarian cyst	

Related Words	Thesaurus	Examples	Own Notes
oophoron (cont'd)	ovary	ovaritis	
opening	dilation ecstasis orifice ostium ostomy patent	cervical dilator vasodilator bronchiectasis cystostomy patent airway	
ophthalmia		ophthalmitis ophthalmologist	
optometry	vision test visual examination	optician optometrist	
orchis	didymus testicle testis	didymitis orchitis testitis testalgia testectomy	

organogenesis	prenatal
	  development
		embryonic
		  development	

orgasm	aphrodisia anaphrodisiac coitus excitement masturbation orgasmic maturity	sexual arousal no sexual arousal onanism	
origin	generic genesis	generic name algogenesis carcinogenesis oncogenesis	
ortho	orthodontics orthogenic orthopedic orthopedics orthopnea orthoptic	orthodontic band orthopsychiatry orthopedic surgery orthopedist orthopsia	

Related Words	Thesaurus	Examples	Own Notes
ortho (cont'd)	orthostatic	orthostatic hypotension	
osteo-	bone	osteoarthritis osteofibrosis osteonecrosis osteophytes	
osteoporosis		bone atrophy	
outgoing	efferent	efferent vessels	
ovulation	menses	ovarian expulsion	

Section P

Related Words	Thesaurus	Examples	Own Notes
pacemaker	cardioverter	defibrillator	
pain	ailment algesia algia dolor dynia migraine pain sore	stomach ailment sensitivity to pain neuralgia psychogenic pain proctodynia migraine headache chronic pain pain threshold sore throat	
pain control	anesthesia nerve block painkiller palliation sedation	analgesics narcotic analgesics palliative care	
paleness	pallor		
palpitate	beat palpitation pulse	heartbeat pulsation	
palsy	numbness palsy paralysis paraplegia polio stupefaction	cerebral palsy flaccid paralysis spastic paralysis diplegia hemiplegia peripheral paraplegia poliomyelitis	
pandemic	endemic epidemic pandemic	endemic goiter endemiology	

Related Words	Thesaurus	Examples	Own Notes
panesthesia	cenesthesia panesthesia	cenesthesis	
panic	phobia	panic attack panic disorder anxiety disorder	
Pap smear test	Pap test	cervical cancer test	
papilla	nipple papilla teat (obsolete)	papillitis papilloma nipple	
papule	pimple	papulation	
paralyze	cripple demoralize hemiplegia numbness paralysis paresis paresthesis	paraplegia	
paramedic	emergency medical		
paranoia	delirium paranoia paranoid phreno- phrenopathy psychosis schizophrenia	mental confusion hallucinatory paranoia alcoholic paranoia paranoid disorder related to the mind	
paraplegia	hemiplegia -plegic	psychoplegic	
parasite	bloodsucker commensal leech symbiont		

Related Words	Thesaurus	Examples	Own Notes
parosmia	anosmia parosmia	cacosmia	
paroxysmal	convulsion seizure spasm sudden attack transient	transient attack	
parturition	delivery partus	giving birth	
passive tremor	Parkinson's disease resting tremor		
pasteurize	disinfect sterilize		
pathology	morbid physiology pathogenesis pathophysiology pathosis	diseased condition	
penetrate	diffuse effusion infiltrate osmosis permeate pervade seep	diffusibility pleural effusion infiltration permeable pervasion	
perceptible	cognizable observable sensible tangible	cognition sensibility	
percussion	impact impulse strike		
perforate	pierce punch	perforation	

Comprehensive Medical Thesaurus

Related Words	Thesaurus	Examples	Own Notes
perineotomy	episiotomy		
periodontium	parodental parodontium periodontal disease periodontia periodontoclasia periodontosis	parodentist parodontitis gumboil periodontitis permanent teeth damage periodental disease	
periosteum	bone vascular membrane		
peritoneum	abdominal membrane	peritonitis	
pertussis	whooping cough		
phobia	acrophobia agoraphobia erythophobia fear-tension syndrome		
phrenic	diaphragm mind phrenic nerve neurosis	phrenitis phrenodynia phrenopathy schizophrenia	
pilar cyst	sebaceous cyst		
pimple	acne comedo papule	papulation	
pineal body	epiphysis cerebri pineal gland		
pituitary	hypophysis	hypophysis gland	
pivot joint	articulation gliding joint		

Related Words	Thesaurus	Examples	Own Notes
pivot joint (cont'd)	hinge joint socket joint trochoid		
placenta	chorion placenta previta	choriocarcinoma placentitis placentoma placenta orevita	
plague	Bacillus fleas pesticide poisoning	bubonic plague pneumonic plague white plague	
plaque	atherosclerosis caries plaque	dental caries dental plaque	
plasma	blood serum plasma plasmapheresis serum	serous fluid plasma cell plasma protein plasma exchange serum sickness	
platelet	thrombocyte		
plethora	erythrocytosis polycythemia	ideopathic blood disorder	
pleura	intercostal pleural pleurisy pleurodynia	pleural effusion pleuralgia	
pneumo	lung pneumocystis pneumoconiosis pneumonectomy pneumonia pneumonitis pneumothorax pulmonary	lung cancer pneumocystosis asbestosis pulmonary edema pulmonary embolism	

COMPREHENSIVE MEDICAL THESAURUS

Related Words	Thesaurus	Examples	Own Notes
pneumo (cont'd)	tuberculosis		
podiatry	podalgia podarthritis podema podiatrist podiatry podium	 foot doctor podology pseudopodium	
poison	Bacillus bacterial bane botulism clostridium endotoxin enterotoxin Escherichia Coli Salmonella toxin venom virus	bacillary bacterial pathogens enterotoxemia E. Coli salmonellosis toxicant venomous virulent	
polio	muscular atrophy polioencephalitis poliomyelitis poliosis		
pollinosis	hay fever		
poor	ana- ano- ataxic cachexia caco- emaciation mal- oligo-	anapepsia anorexia aphasia ataxia ataxic speech cachexy cacochylia cacophony excessive leanness malnutrition oligopepsia	
porphyria	porphrins	erythropoietic	

Related Words	Thesaurus	Examples	Own Notes
porphyria (cont'd)		hepatic porphyria porphyrinuria	
pregnancy	childbearing cyesis gestation maternity pregnancy	celiocyesis gestation age ectopic pregnancy	
precocious	premature	precocity	
presby	presbyatrics geriatrics	presbycusis presbyopia	
proct	anal proct rectum rectus	anal atresia proctalgia rectalgia rectus muscle	
produce	generate proliferate propagate	proliferation propagation	
propagate	disseminate		
proptosis	bulging ptosis	gastric ptosis	
prophylactic	preventive prophylaxis vaccine		
prostate	prostalgia prostatic growth prostato-	prostatauxe prostatic hyperplasia prostatic hypertrophy prostatomegaly	
prosthesis	prosthetic	prosthetist prosthetic dentistry prosthodontia	

Related Words	Thesaurus	Examples	Own Notes
proteinuria	albuminuria		
psychic	mind psychiatry psychic contagion	psychic force psychoanalyst psychic infection	

psychopath	antisocial man
	
	psychotic
	psychosexual
	
	sociopath
		psychopathic
		  personality
		psychotic disorder
		psychosexual
		  disorder
		sociopathy (obsolete)	

psychosis	mental disorder paranoia schizophrenia	psychoneurosis alcoholic psychosis bipolar disorder mental disorder	
pubic	genitals genitalia pubis	pubic region genital reflex pubic bones	
pudendum	episio- perineal perineum vulva vulvar vulvovaginal	episiotomy perineotomy external genitalia vulvitis vulvectomy vulvovaginitis	
pulse	pulsus paradoxus rythmic beating sphygmo-	paradoxical pulse sphygmogram sphygmometer	
purpura	erythematosa purpura fulminans purpura paulosa purpura urticans senile purpura		

Related Words	Thesaurus	Examples	Own Notes
pus	abscess cerumen empyema excretion expectorant expectorate exudate furuncle phlegm purulent sputum	pulmonary abscess earwax pleural empyema empyema thoracis excrement mucolytic ear furuncle cellular debris	
pyelo	pelvis kidney	pyelograph pyelonephritis	
pygo	buttocks	pygomelus	
pyogenic	purulent pye- pyo- pyoderma pyogenic pyopoietic pyorrhea pyosis suppurative	purulent edema pyemesis pyemia pyesis pyometritis pyonephritis pyo-ovarium pyopericarditis impetigo pyogenic bacteria pyorrhea alveolaris pyotorrhea pyothorax suppurative otitis	

Section Q

Related Words	Thesaurus	Examples	Own Notes
Q fever	febris	Australian Q fever	
quack	charlatan quack quackery	charlatanic quack doctor	
quarantine	confinement detention exclusion isolation quarantine seclusion		
quasi	apparent approximate pseudo quasi	pseudoarthritis pseudocyesis pseudofracture quasi blend quasi reflex	
queer	strange		
quick	sensitive tachy	tachycardia tachyrhythmia tachylalia	
quinsy	peritonsillar abscess quinsy	tonsillitis	
quiver	quaver quiver shake shiver shudder tremble tremor	quavery quivering continuous tremor intention tremor	
Q wave	cardiac cycle electrocardiogram	QRS complex	

Section R

Related Words	Thesaurus	Examples	Own Notes
ramus	branch ramification ramus	secretory branch ramus bronchalis	
range	limit range scope	range of motion	

reaction	activator
	agglutination
	
	allergy
	anaphylaxis
	hypersensitive
	  reaction
	reflex
	sensibility
		motor neuron
		spontaneous
		  agglutination
		allergic reaction
		anaphylactic shock
		conditioned reflexes
		
		inborn reflex	

receptacle	capsule cell cyst follicle paunch (obsolete) pouch receiver receptor sac saccule ventricle vesicle	capsula cell division cystic carcinoma cystic fibroma follicular cyst stomach sensor cul-de-sac saccus ventricle of the heart saclike structure	
recovery	recuperation relief remedy remission restoration suspension		

Comprehensive Medical Thesaurus

Related Words	Thesaurus	Examples	Own Notes
rectitis	proctitis		
rectocele	proctocele		
rectoscope	proctoscope		
rectotomy	proctotomy		
recurrence	recidivation (obsolete) recrudescent relapse	revert return of symptom	
relieve	alleviate release		
rem	sievert		
remission	diminution	disappearance of symptom	
removal	dialysis emesis enervation excision exclusion expel pheresis	hemodialysis vomitus removal of a nerve vomit apheresis plasmapheresis	
renal calculus	kidney stone nephritic calculus		
respiration	breathing respiration respirator	artificial respiration nebulizer	
respiratory	spinogram spinometry	spirometer	
rhinal	rhinitis rhinopathy sinusitis	inflamed nostril	

Related Words	Thesaurus	Examples	Own Notes
rhinolalia	rhinophonia		
rhinorrhagia	epistaxis nosebleed		
rheumatic	ankylosing ankylosis dermatomyositis fibromyalgia polymyalgia polymyositis rheumatoid rheumatic	ankylosing spondylitis rheumatoid arthritis rheumatism rheumatic arthritis rheumatic pericarditis	
rima	cleft fissure laceration rima glottis rima oris	cleft palate fissura pudendi perineal laceration rima glottidis	
-rrhea	diarrhea hemorrhage rhinorrhea		
rumination	backward flow regurgitation	second chewing aortic regurgitation	
rump (obsolete)	buttocks nates pygo	pygopagus	
rupture	clasia diverticulum hernia hiatus perforate puncture rupture	aortoclasia diverticulosis abdominal hernia hiatus hernia perforation intervertebral ruptured disc	

Section S

Related Words	Thesaurus	Examples	Own Notes
saccule	saccular sacculus saccus vesica vesicle	saccular aneurysm alveolar sac vesical calculus	
sadism	algolagnia pedophilia sadism	sexual perversion molesting children sexual abuse	
saliva	Bartholin's duct parotid duct	salivary duct salivary gland	
salping	fallopian tube	salpingectomy salpingotomy	
salpinx		auditory salpinx	
sane	normal sanity soundness		
sarco-	sarcoid sarcoidosis sarcoma	flesh sarcomatosis	
scab	eschar escharosis scab	eschartomy scabies	
scapula	shoulder blade scapulohumeral	scapulohumeral reflex	
scarlet fever	scarlatina		
schizo	division schizocaria		

Related Words	Thesaurus	Examples	Own Notes
schizo (cont'd)	schizocephalia schizocyte schizogenesis split	splitting	
schizophrenia	paranoia schizoid schizophasia schizotypal	schizoid personality word salad	
sciatica	back pain sciatic	disk prolapse sciatic nerve	
scirrhoid	scirrhoma scirrhous scirrhus	scirrhous carcinoma	
sclera	sclera sclerectomy scleritis sclerotomy	sclerotitis	
sclerose	catalepsy sclerocataracta sclerocornea scleroderma scleroma sclerosis sclerostenosis sclerosing solution	cataleptic arterial sclerosis atherosclerosis sclerotherapy stopping hemorrhage	
scoliosis	kyphoscoliosis kyphosis lordosis spinal curvature		
scrobiculous	pit pock	pockmarks	
scurvy	ascorbic acid disorder scorbutus		

COMPREHENSIVE MEDICAL THESAURUS

Related Words	Thesaurus	Examples	Own Notes
seizure	convulsion focal seizure grand mal seizure	epilepsy motor seizure petit mal seizure	
semen	germ seed seminal fluid seminales sperm	germination seminal vesicle seminal vesiculitis vesicula seminales spermatocyst	
senile	aging gera geriatrics gero presby senescence senile	gerantotherapy geriatrician geropsychology presbycardia senescent senile cataract senile delirium senile involution senile psychosis senile warts	
sensate	orgasm sensate sensation stimulation	orgasmic maturity sensate focus technique sexual stimulation	
sensitivity	allergic anaphilactic atopic	atopic asthma	
sensory apraxia	abasia amnestic apraxia apraxia of speech motor apraxia	paralytic abasia	
separation anxiety		anxiety neurosis	
septic arthritis	bacterial arthritis septic bursitis		

Related Words	Thesaurus	Examples	Own Notes
septum	atrium septum diaphragm interseptum	cordis septum diaphragmalgia	
serous	serology serous fluid serosanguinous serum serum sickness serum albumin serous membrane serotonin serosynovitis	serologist serologic diagnosis serum hepatitis immunologic disorder protein in blood serosa serositis	
sex	coitus genitalia lust onanism orgasm sadism sensate sex sexual sexual reflex STD	intercourse masturbation sexual climax sexual perversion delayed sensation sex chromosome sexual dysfunction genital reflex sexually transmitted disease	
shigellosis	bacillary dysentery		
shingles	herpes, genital herpes simplex herpes zoster	herpes sexualis herpes gestation	
shoulder	acromion scapular shoulder blade	scapulalgia	
sialorrhea	drool ptyalis ptyalorrhea ptyalosis saliva	drooling excessive salivation ptyalism salivation	

Related Words	Thesaurus	Examples	Own Notes
sialorrhea (cont'd)	sialogogue sialoma	sialosis	
sidero	homochromatosis iron deficiency anemia iron metabolism siderocyte sideropenia siderosis		
sitology	nutrition sito sitosterol sitotherapy threpology	food, nutrition sitology	

skin	corium
	cortex
	
	cutaneous
	
	cuticle
	cutis
	cutis marmorata
	derma
	dermato
	dermis
	epidermis
	epithelium
	
	integument
	
	sebaceous
	
	sebum
		
		outer layer
		renal cortex
		percutaneous
		subcutaneous
		transcutaneous
		cuticular
		cutis laxa
		livedo
		dermal
		dermatology
		
		squamous
		  epithelium
		integumentary
		  system
		oil-secreting
		  skin
		oily secretion	

skin disorders	atopic eczema carcinoma cutaneous cutitis	 squamous cell carcinoma cutaneous papilloma	

Related Words	Thesaurus	Examples	Own Notes
skin disorders (cont'd)	cutis laxa dermatitis dermatocyst dermatoma keratosis leiodermia leiomyoma lesion livedo melanoma prurigo pruritus scleroderma shingles skin cancer skin grafting	loose skin melanoma senile keratosis smooth skin leiomyoma cutis livedo reticularis skin cancer prurigo vulgaris pruritus cutaneous chicken pox, varicella herpes genitalis herpes simplex herpes zoster melanoma skin implant	
slaver	drivel saliva		
sleep disorder	apnea hypnosis lethargy narcolepsy nightmare sleep terror sleepwalking sleepless somnolent soporific soporose (obsolete)	sleep apnea pavor nocturnus somnambulism noctambulism anhypnia somniferous deep sleep comatose	
smell badly	cacosmia osmidrosis stench stink	kakosmia	
sneezing	sternutation	sternutatory	

Related Words	Thesaurus	Examples	Own Notes
sobriety	moderation restrain sobriety temperance	field sobriety test	

spasmophilia	convulsive
	myoclonic
	paroxysm
	paroxysmal
	
	seizure
	spasm
	spasmatic
	spasmodic
	
	spasmogen
	spasmophilia
	
	spastic
		tetany convulsion
		myoclonus
		
		paroxysmal
		  tachycardia
		
		spasmodermia
		gastrospasm
		spasmodic
		  dysphonia
		
		spasmodic
		  tendency
		spastic bladder
		reflex bladder	

spermatic duct	testicular duct vas deferens	vasectomy	
spina bifida	spinal cord disorder spina bifida cystica spina bifida occulta	congenital spinal disorder meningocele myelocele	
spinal column	dorsal column spine spondylo vertebra vertebral	dorsalgia spinitis spondylodynia vertebra joint vertebral artery	
spinal cord	funiculus marrow medulla	funiculitis bone marrow medullitis	
spiro	spirochete (spiral bacterium)	Bacillus	

Related Words	Thesaurus	Examples	Own Notes
spiro (cont'd)	spiro	spirogram spirometer	
spittle	drooling ptyalin saliva sialorrhea	drooly ptyalosis	
splancho	internal organ splanchna splanchnic splanchno viscera viscus	splanchnic nerve splanchnocele splanchnodynia	
spondyl	spina spinal column spondyl spondylo vertebra vertebro	spinal caries spondylitis spondylosis vertebral canal vertebrocostal	
spore	sporo sporoblast sporogenesis sporulation	sporocyst	
sprain	joint sprain	ligament sprain tendon sprain	
stammer	angophrasia aphasia dysphemia stuttering	stammering	
steato	lipa lipo lipoid steatitis steato	lipemia lipofibroma liposarcoma steatoma	
sthenia	strength	eusthenia	

Related Words	Thesaurus	Examples	Own Notes
steno	contraction emaciation narrowing steno stricture	tonic contraction excessive leanness stenocardia stenosis constriction	
stenosis	coarctation	coarctation of aorta pyroric stenosis vaginal stenosis vascular stenosis	
sterilization	cystectomy hysterectomy tubal ligation tubectomy vasectomy		
sterno	chest sternum stetho	chest X-ray sternocostal stethomytis stethoscope	
sterol	calciferol cholesterol ergosterol viosterol	vitamin D_2	
stomach	gastric paunch stomach	gastritis stomachalgia	
stone	calculus crystal gastrolith inolith lithiasis litho- lithotrity	prostatic calculus crystallization cholelithiasis lithogenesis litholysis lithotomy lithotriptor	
stop	abort	habitual abortion	

Related Words	Thesaurus	Examples	Own Notes

stop (cont'd)	block
	immune
	inhibit
	miscarry
	nerve block
	
	prevent
	
	restrain
	suppress
	vaccination
		induced abortion
		spontaneous
		  abortion
		voluntary abortion
		blocking antibody
		artificial immunity
		inhibitor
		missed abortion
		nerve block
		  anesthesia
		preventive care
		prophylaxis
		restraint
		suppressor	

strains	distortions orthodontic prosthodontic	musculoskeletal strain orthodontic headgear cantilever bridge	
strangulation	constriction	constricting ring intestinal strangulation	
stratum	layer stratum basale stratum corneum	horny layer	

strep throat	choking
	sore throat
	strep throat
	streptococcal
	  angina
	streptococcal
	  cellulitis
	streptococcal
	  pneumonia
		infected pharynx	

stricture	stenosis	aortic stenosis	
stroke	blood stroke cerebral infarction cerebrovascular	cerebral hemorrhage	

Comprehensive Medical Thesaurus

Related Words	Thesaurus	Examples	Own Notes
stroke (cont'd)	accident heat stroke	sun stroke	
stupor	anergic stupor coma epileptic stupor lethargy stunning senselessness unconscious	AIDS due to lack of activity delusion stupor	
stye (or sty)	hordeolum chalazion		
styptic	astringent control bleeding	local tightening	
succus	juice sap	juicy sappy succulence	
suck	suckle suckling	breast-feed suckling reflex	
sudor	sudorific sweat	sudoresis sudorrhea sudation	
sugar	diabetes glucose glycerol glycogen sweet		
sulcus	fissure sulcus vallecula valley	lateral fissure central sulcus sulcus cerebri vallecula cerebella vallecula cordis	
supine	supination	face-up position	

Related Words	Thesaurus	Examples	Own Notes
supine (cont'd)	supine hypotension supine position	vena caval syndrome	
swallow	deglutition		
sweat gland	apocrine gland sebaceous gland sudoriferous gland	sebaceous crypt	
swelling	boil edema emphysema lipoma tumor	cardiac edema neoplasm	
swoon	faint stun syncope	stunning syncopal attack	
synovial	synovia synovial synovial bursa synovial membrane synovial tendon sheath	synovial fluid synovial joint	

synovial problems	synovial
	  chondroma
	synovial
	  inflammation
		synovial
		  chondromatosis
		synovitis	

syphilis	lues syphillis	syphilitic aortitis	

Section T

Related Words	Thesaurus	Examples	Own Notes
tabes	tabescent tiresome wasting weariness	tabes dorsalis wasting disease	
taboo	forbid prohibit suppress	prohibited article	
taenia	flatworm parasitic taeniasis tapeworm	taenia saginata parasitic glossitis tapeworm infection beef tapeworm	
Tamoxifen	antiestrogen hormone breast cancer drug		
tarsal bone	astragalus calcaneus cuboid hallux talus tarso- tarsus	heel bone cuboidal tarsal bone big toe anklebone tarsalgia edge of the foot anklebone	
T cell	helper cell lymphocyte	suppressor T cell	
tear duct	excretory duct lacrimal duct nasolacrimal duct		
telomere	enzyme	antiaging chromosome	

Related Words	Thesaurus	Examples	Own Notes
telomere (cont'd)	repaired DNA telomere	telomerase enzyme DNA strand division	
tendon	fibrous band ligament tendon teno-	Achilles tendon tendonplastic tendon reflex tenodynia tenonitis tenosynovitis tenotomy	
teras	freak monster prodigy teratism teratogenesis teratoid	teratosis teratogeny teratoma	
terminology	etymology glossology lingo nomenclature term	etymological study linguistics technical term	
terror	fear panic pavor terror	fear-tension syndrome panic terror pavor nocturia terrify	
testis	didym orchid (obsolete) orchis testicle testis	didymus didymitis orchidectomy (obsolete) orchiditis (obsolete) orchiectomy orchitis testicular duct vas deferens testicular vein male gonads	

Related Words	Thesaurus	Examples	Own Notes
testosterone	androgenic hormone anabolic steroid testosterone derivative		
thigh	femoral femur thigh	thighbone thigh joint	
thoraco	chest thoracoabdominal thoracentesis thoraco thorax	chest X-ray exam thoracocentesis thoracodynia	
throat	laryngeal larynx pharynx throat	laryngitis the organ of voice pharyngitis sore throat	
throb	beat palpitate pulsate throbbing	heartbeat palpitation	
thrombo	blood clot embolism thrombo thrombolytics thrombosis thrombus	pulmonary embolism thromboembolism clot busters cardiac thrombosis agonal thrombus	
thrush	candidiasis	oral candidiasis	
thyroxine	thyrotropic hormone		
tinea	athlete's foot jock itch tinea	fungal skin disease tinea cruris ringworm tinea capitis	

Related Words	Thesaurus	Examples	Own Notes
toco	birth delivery labor toco	tocomania	
toenail	unguis	nail	
tongue	glossal glosso lingua lingual tongue-tie	glossitis glossodynia lingual lingual frenum ankyloglossia	
tonic	invigorating stimulating tone tonus tonia tonic tonicity	invigoration balanced tension strong tension hypertonia cardiac tonic muscle contraction quality of tone	
topical	local surface topo	local anesthesia surface anesthesia toponarcosis	
torpid	dormant lethargic numbness stagnant torpid torpor	lethargy sluggish torpidity inactivity	
toxin	botulism carbon monoxide dioxin poison toxicant toxicity toxin toxoid toxolysin	porphyria cutanea tarda poisonous toxicology vaccine	

Related Words	Thesaurus	Examples	Own Notes
toxin (cont'd)	vaccine venom virulence virus	virulent parasitic microorganism	
trachea	primary bronchus windpipe	tracheitis trachalgia	
tranquilizer	antipsychotic oxazepam pacify sedate tranquilizer	Serax (trade name) pacifier	
transfection	infection metastasis migrate transmission	migratory pain transmit	
transfer	transfusion transplant transposition transposon transsexual	blood transfusion transfer of genes	
transpose	sex change transvestism		
trauma	disruptive injury traumatic	traumatic delirium	
tremble	palsy paralysis paralytic Parkinson's disease quiver shaking shudder tremble tremor	shaking palsy cerebral paralysis facial paralysis intention tremor involuntary tremor	

Related Words	Thesaurus	Examples	Own Notes
tricho-	hair trichogen trichoid tricoma trichonosis trichopathy trichorrhea trichotillomania	trichogenous trichologia trichomania	
troph	autotroph nourishment nutrient sitology troph-	embryotroph nutrition threpology trophology trophtherapy	
tubal	tubal abortion tubal ligation tubectomy vasectomy	tubal pregnancy sterilization	
tubercle	tuberculin tuberculoma tuberculosis, TB	TB BCG vaccine	
tuberculum	tuberosis tuberosity tuberous sclerosis		
tumor	celioma encephaloma fibroadenoma fibroid hamartoma neoplasma neoplastic onco— oncovirus	celioncus fibroma tumorlike mass oncology oncofetal protein oncogenesis	
typhlo-	cecum blind (gut)	cecotomy typhlotomy typhlolexia	
typhoid fever	enteric fever typhoid	epidemic typhus typhus vaccine	

Section U

Related Words	Thesaurus	Examples	Own Notes
umbilicus	bellybutton navel omphal umbilical	omphalocele umbilical hernia	
unconscious	coma faint stun swoon syncope		
unquis	nail		
ureter	ureter urethra urinary	ureterolith urethrostomy urinary calculus	
urination	micturition urine urogenital	micturate urinoscopy genitourinary	
urticaria	hives		
urogram	pyelogram	urinary tract	
uterus	hyster hystero metra metria metro uterine womb	hysteralgia hysterocyesis metralgia metritis metrodynia uteritis uterus	

Section V

Related Words	Thesaurus	Examples	Own Notes
vaginal	colpopathy vaginal	colpodynia vaginitis	
varicella	chicken pox		
varices	aneurysm dilated vein varices vena veno-	dilated vessel distended vein varicosis varicoectomy vena cava venotomy	
vas	varix vas vasal vaso vein vena cava venule	varicose vein blood vessel lymph spermatoza vas deferens vasculitis vasectomy vasoconstriction vasodilation venipuncture venotomy venular	
vasospastic	angina vasoconstriction vasospasm	chest pain angiospasm	
vasovagal	vasodepressor syncope vasovagal attack	 vasovagal syncope	
vein	phlebo varicose	phlebogram phlebotomy varicosis	

Related Words	Thesaurus	Examples	Own Notes
vein (cont'd)	vena veni veno	varicose aneurysm varicotomy vena cava venectasis venipuncture venotomy	
ventral	abdominal ventral	abdominal hernia ventral hernia	
ventricle	belly ventro	small cavity ventrodorsal	
verruca	verruca plana verruca vulgaris	flat wart	
vertigo	dizziness		
vesicle	small bladder	blister	
vesicle calculus	cystolith	bladder stone	
vesicle reflex	micturition reflex urinate sensation		
vessel	angio artery coronary phleb vas or vasa vascular vaso vessel	angioma pulmonary artery coronary thrombosis phlebotomy vessel (blood) neovascularization vasodilation vessel occlusion	

virion	bacterium
	
	plasmid
	
	poison
	viral
	viro
		parasitic
		  microorganism
		bacterial
		  chromosome
		
		viral infection
		virocytes	

Related Words	Thesaurus	Examples	Own Notes
viron (cont'd)	viroid virulent virus virustatic	transposon virulence adenovirus antipropagation	

viscera	viscus
	enteron
	splanchnic
	visceral
	
	viscerate
		internal organ
		splanchnocele
		visceral nervous
		  system
		involuntary
		  nervous system
		eviscerate	

vitreous humor	corpus vitreum vitreous membrane	vitreous body	
vocal	aphasia stammer vocal cords	dysphemia vocal folds	
voluntary	elective voluntary	elective abortion voluntary abortion	
voluntary muscle	skeletal muscle	striated muscle striated fibers	

volvulus	bowel twisting
	volvulus
	  neonatorum
		intestinal
		  obstruction	

vomit	emesis regurgitate	regurgitation	

Section W

Related Words	Thesaurus	Examples	Own Notes
waist	lumbar lumbar nerves	loin nerves in the lumbar spinal region	
wall	cortex diaphragm methothelium mural	renal cortex mural thrombus of the heart	
warts	verruca warts	verruca vulgaris genital warts	
wash	cleansing lavage purge	gastric lavage	
wax	cerumen earwax grease tallow	sebum of the skin	
weak	debility emaciate frailty feebleness infirmity prostrate	emaciation infirmary prostration	
wheezing	asthma bronchitis		
whiplash	neck injury		
windpipe	larynx tracheo	tracheomalacia tracheotomy	
worsen	aggravate	aggravation	

Section X

Related Words	Thesaurus	Examples	Own Notes
X-chromosome	sex chromosome	X-X chromosome X-Y chromosome	
xanchromatic	jaune lutein xanchromia xanth yellowish	jaundice luteoma hemoglobin breakdown xanthemia xanthous race	
xanthine	xanthic xanthine derivative icterus luteal	yellowish xanthinuria jaundice luteoma	
xanthoma	xanthosis	xanthomatosis	
xantho-	xanthochromic xanthoma xanthopsia xanthosis xanthous	xanthochromia xanthomatosis	
xeno	hetero strange xeno-	heterodermic heterograft xenogenesis xenograft xenoparasite xenophobia xenophonia	
xero	dry xeransis xero xero	dry catarrh dry cough dryness xeransia xerochilia xeroderma xerophthalmia xeroradiography xerostomia	

Section Y

Related Words	Thesaurus	Examples	Own Notes
yawn	gape yawning weariness		
yaws	buba frambesia yaws	bouba spirochete infection	
yeast	ferment yeast	diastolic ferment digestive ferment pathological yeast	
yellow disease	cirrhosis luteoma icterus yellow cartilage yellow fever	biliary cirrhosis fatty cirrhosis pregnancy luteoma jaundice elastic cartilage yellow fever vaccine	
yogurt	curdled milk		
yoke	bond connector link yolk	bondage linkage yolk sac yolk stalk	
yolk	placenta umbilical cord	nutritive membrane umbilical duct	

Section Z

Related Words	Thesaurus	Examples	Own Notes
zona	zona zone zonesthesia zonula, zonule zonula ciliaris	zona glomerulosa zona reticularis zone therapy girdle sensation zonula ciliaris zonule of Zinn zonulitis	
zygote	blastocyst blastogenesis fertilization gametes gametogenesis zygogenesis zygosis zygosity zygosperm zygote	sexual reproduction monozygosity zygospore blastocyst	
zymoma	chief cell enzyme ferment zymogen zymology zymolysis zymosis zymotic	zymogenic cell fermentation zymogenesis zymotic disease	
zymophyte	zymocyte zymogenic	zymogene	

PART II

Analytical Study

CHAPTER 1

ANALYSIS OF STRUCTURE AND MEDICAL MODIFIERS

A) Structural Analysis of Expanding Terminology

Example 1: "Erythroderm" -------------- Red-skin disease.

This is an example of "Compound Terminology" with a simple prefix "Erythro."

Erythro ---------------- Prefix meaning "red."

derma ----------------- Stem meaning "skin."

Example 2: "Erythema Nodosum" ------------ Red-skin disease at the node.

Erythema is an example of "Compound Terminology" with a prefix meaning also red although the spelling is different.

"Erythema Nodosum" is an example of "Combined Terminology."

Erythema ------------- Main word

Nodosum ------------- Post modifier to indicate the location of the body.

This is an example in which a modifier is placed after the main word to make a "Combined Terminology."

Example 3: "Myocarditis" ---------------- An inflammation of heart muscle.

This is an example of "Complex Compound Terminology" with a prefix "Myo" meaning "Muscle" and a suffix "itis" meaning "inflammation."

Example 4: Cardiomyopathy" --------------- Heart muscle failure.

"Cardiomyopathy" is also an example of "Complex Compound Terminology" with three polysyllabic words.

Cardio ----------------- Prefix meaning "heart."

myo -------------------- Main stem meaning "muscle."

pathy ------------------ Suffix meaning "illness."

Example 5: "Cerebral Infarction" (   ) Stroke (   )

This is commonly called "stroke" by people in general. The loss of blood flow and oxygen to a part of the brain is the most serious trouble.

The structure of terminology is similar to Example 6, except the modifier is not a compound modifier as in Example 6, but a simple modifier.

Example 6: "Myocardial Infarction" ----------------------- Heart attack

This is an example of "Combined Terminology" with a compound modifier placed before the main word "infarction." (Compare with Example 2.)

"Myo" is again a prefix attached to the compound modifier "myocardial."

"Myocardial" ------- Compound modifier, meaning "heart muscle."
"Infarction" --------- Main word, meaning loss of blood flow which causes heart tissue failure.

Table 1: Structural Analysis

Types	Structural Analysis	Example No.
Simple Compound	Prefix + Stem	1
Complex Compound	Prefix + (Stem + Suffix)	3
Same		4
Combined Terminology	Simple modifier + Main word	5
	Compound Modifier + Main word	6
Same	Compound Terminology + Postmodifier	2

Meaning of Examples

Example 1:   Erythroderma

Example 2:   Erythema Nodosum

Example 3:   Myocarditis

Example 4:   Cardiomyopathy

Example 5:   Cerebral Infarction

Example 6:   Myocardial Infarction

B) Types of Compound Terminology

Table 2 Examples of Simple Compound Terminology

Simple Compound	Meaning of examples
Angiography	
Angioplasty	
Arteriosclerosis	
Chondrosarcoma	
Choriocarcinoma	
Gastrospasm	
Fibroadenoma	
Hemangioma	
Lymphangioma	
Opthalmoplegia	
Poliomyelitis	

Table 3 Examples of Complex Compound Terminology

Complex Compound	Meaning of examples
Cardiomyopathy	
Cholecystectomy	
Cholelithiasis	
Chorioretinopathy	

C) Types of <u>Combined</u> Terminology

Adjective modifiers are used with the combined terminology. These modifiers are placed either before or after the compound nouns, namely regular adjective or reversed postadjective.

For the sake of linguistic study, the modifiers are classified as follows in this book:

Table 4: Simple <u>characteristic</u> a) modifiers

Table 5: <u>Complex</u> b) characteristic modifiers

Table 6: Simple <u>body</u> c) modifiers

Table 7: Compound body modifiers

Explanation of terms used above:

a) "Characteristic" means characteristics of diseases or disorders.

b) "Complex" means stem plus prefix or suffix (Chapter 1, b, Table 3).

c) "Body" means one or two locations of the body.

Table 4
Examples of Simple Characteristic Modifiers

Modifiers	Meanings	Examples	Meaning of Examples
Acquired		<u>Acquired</u> immunity	
Acute		<u>Acute</u> rhinitis	
Afferent		<u>Afferent</u> sensory	
Allergic		<u>Allergic</u> rhinitis	
Anemic		<u>Anemic</u> anoxia	
Anterior		<u>Anterior</u> Achilles tendons	
Ataxic		<u>Ataxic</u> aphasia	

Comprehensive Medical Thesaurus

Modifiers	Meanings	Examples	Meaning of Examples
Atopic		<u>Atopic</u>m dermatitis	
Bacterial		<u>Bacterial</u> pneumonia	
Benign		<u>Benign</u> tumor	
Brady		<u>Brady</u>cardia	
Catatonic		<u>Catatonic</u> excitement	
Chronic		<u>Chronic</u> pharyngitis	
Congenital		<u>Congenital</u> myopathy	
Dendrite		<u>Dendrite</u> nerve	
Dextro		<u>Dextro</u>cardia	
Dissecting		<u>Dissecting</u> aneurysm	
Efferent		<u>Efferent</u> nerve	
Epidemic		<u>Epidemic</u> AIDS	
Frontal		<u>Frontal</u> lobe	
Habitual		<u>Habitual</u> abortion	
Hereditary		<u>Hereditary</u> ataxia	
Idiopathic		<u>Idiopathic</u> osteonecrosis	
Insidious		<u>Insidious</u> AIDS	
Malignant		<u>Malignant</u> lymphoma	
Melano		<u>Melano</u>sarcoma	
Metastic		<u>Metastic</u> cancer	
Multiple		<u>Multiple</u> sclerosis	

Modifiers	Meanings	Examples	Meaning of Examples
Oppotunistic		Oppotunistic infections	
Osmatic		Osmatic axillae	
Paroxismal		Paroxysmal tachycardia	
Peripheral		Peripheral nerve	
Pernicious		Pernicious anemia	
Prodromal		Prodromal labor	
Progressive		Progressive dystrophy	
Prolific		Prolific source	
Proximal		Proximal tubules	
Purulent		Purulent meningitis	
Pyogenic		Pyogenic spondylitis	
Rheumatoid		Rheumatoid arthritis	
Senile		Senile dementia	
Stress		Stress incontinence	
Suppurative		Suppurative boil	
Sympathetic		Sympathetic dystrophy	
Symptomatic		Symptomatic benign prostatauxe	
Systemic		Systemic sclerosis	
Topical		Topical anesthetics	
Transient		Transient attack	
Ulcerative		Ulcerative colitis	

Table 4A
Adjective by Location in the Body

Modifiers	Meanings	Examples	Meaning of Examples
Anterior		Anterior mediastinum	
Dorsal		Dorsal root system	
Lateral		Lateral nerve tract	
Medial		Medial lemniscus	
Mediolateral		Mediolateral incision*	
Posterior		Posterior artery	
Ventral		Ventral nerve tract	
Visceral		Visceral nervous system	

*Episiotomy

Table 5
Example of Complex Characteristic Modifiers

Modifiers	Examples	
cytochemical	cytochemical assay	
diffusing capacity	diffusing capacity of lungs	
hypersensitivity	hypersensitivity pneumonia	
hypertensive	hypertensive encephalopathy	
hypertonic	hypertonic uterine contraction	

Table 6
Example of Simple Body Modifiers

Modifiers	Examples
abdominal	abdominal respiration
aortic	aortic stenosis
arterial	arterial thrombosis
articular	articular contracture
cartilaginous	cartilaginous metaplasia
cerebral	cerebral hemorrhage
cervical	cervical spondylosis
corneal	corneal reflex
cutaneous	cutaneous anaphylaxis
dental	dental hemorrhage
diabetic	diabetic coma
diagnostic	diagnostic anesthesia
duodenal	duodenal ulcer
esophageal	esophageal stenosis
gastric	gastric spasm
laryngeal	laryngeal spasm
mitral	mitral stenosis
muscular	muscular peristalsis
parietal	parietal peritoneum
pectoral	pectoral muscle

Table 6
Example of Simple Body Modifiers (continued)

Modifiers	Examples	
prostatic	prostatic cancer	
pulmonary	pulmonary infarction	
systemic	systemic circulation	
venous	venous thrombosis	

Table 7
Examples of Compound Body Modifiers

Modifiers	Examples	
cerebrospinal	cerebrospinal fluid	
chondroblast	chondroblastoma	
dentoalveolar	dentoalveolar cyst	
epidermal	epidermal nevus	
esophagobronchial	esophagobronchial fistula	
myocardial	myocardial infarction	
spinocerebellar	spinocerebellar degeneration	

Table 8
Examples of Reversed Modifiers or Post Modifiers

Modifiers	Examples	
axillae	osmidrosis axillae	
basalis	decidua basalis	
congenita	atrichia congenita	
contagiosa	impetigo contagiosa	
deformans	spondylitis deformans	
media	otitis media	
nervosa	anorexia nervosa	
parietalis	decidua parietalis	
pulmonale	cor pulmonale	
sebaceous	nevus sebaceous	
sicca	rhinitis sicca	

CHAPTER 2

ETYMOLOGY OF MEDICAL COMPOUND TERMINOLOGY

Many medical terminologies are based on either Latin or Greek languages. The etymology is not the object of writing this book. However, it is important to study some of even obsolete references.[1]

<u>Examples of Greek Origin</u>

Greek Base	Meanings
Hyster	Uterus, Womb, Hysterical*

"Hysterical" behavior has been observed mostly in women.

Compound Terminology	Meaning	Compound Terminology	Meaning
Hyster-ectomy		**Hyster**-esis	
Hyster-ic Neurosis		**Hyster**-ic	
Hyster-o-id		**Hyster**-o-scopy	

---

[1] Donald M. Ayers and Thomas D. Worthen, "English Words from Latin and Greek Elements," Second Edition, by The University of Arizona Press, Tucson, 1986.

Greek Base	Meanings
Psych	Mind, soul

Compound Terminology	Meaning	Compound Terminology	Meaning
Psych-o-logy		**Psych**-o-sis	
Psych-o-neur-o-sis		**Psych**-o-tic	
Psych-o-path		**Psych**-o-ana-ly-sis	
Psych-o-path-o-logy		**Psych**-o-somat-ic	

Examples of Greek Prefixes or Stems

Greek Prefixes	English	
angi	vessel	
athr	joint	
cardi	heart	
cephal	head	
chole	bile, gall	
chondr	cartilage	
cranion	cranium	
cyan	blue	
cyst	bladder, sac, bag	
dolich	long	
encephalo	brain	
endo (Endon)	inward, within	

Greek Prefixes	English
enter	intestine
eury	broad, wide
gluco (Glykys)	sweet
hepat	liver
horm (Hormaien)	stimulation
hyster	uterus
leuco (Leukos)	white
lip	fat
mast	breast
melan	black, dark
neuro	nerve
ortho	straight, normal, correct
oste	bone
ot	ear
path	illness
phlebo	phlebogram
platy	broad, flat
prostho	addition, prosthesis
sclero	hard
somat	body
sten	narrow

Greek Prefixes	English	
thromb	clot	
thryo	thymus gland	

Examples of Greek Suffixes

Greek Suffixes	Meanings	Examples	Meaning of Examples
-ectomy	surgical removal	mastectomy	
-emia	blood condition	anemia	
-iasis	diseased condition	lithiasis	
-itis	inflammation	bronchiitis	
-mania, -maniac	mental disorder	kleptomania	
-oma	tumor	hepatoma	
-osis	diseased condition	endometriosis	
-path(y)	diseased condition	hysteropathy	
-plegia	paralysis	paraplegia	
-rrhea	abnormal discharge	diarrhea	
-tomy	incision	hysterotomy	

Latin Base	Meanings
Spir	to breathe

Latin		Latin	
a-**spir**-a-tion		a-**spir**-ate	
con-**spir**-e		ex-**pir**-ate	
re-**spir**-a-tory		per-**spir**-e	
per-**spir**-a-tion		re-**spir**-at-ion	

Latin Base Examples of Non-Medical Meanings

Latin Base		Latin Base	
a-**spir**-ant		a-**spir**-at-ion	
con-**spir**-at-ion		ex-**pir**-at-ion	
in-**spir**-e		tran-**spir**-e	

Examples of Latin Base

Latin Base	Meanings
Firm	firm, strong

Latin Base		Latin Base	
in-**fir**-**mi**-ty		in-**firm**-ary	
con-**firm**-at-ion		af-**firm**-at-ion	
re-af-**firm**-at-ion			

Classification of the Combination of Latin and Greek Origins:

Medical terminology can be divided into five types depending on the combination of origins:

    Type 1: (Latin + Latin)   Compound Terminology

    Type 2: (Latin + Greek)   Compound Terminology

    Type 3: (Latin + Greek Compound)   Combination Terminology

    Type 4: (Greek + Latin)   Compound Terminology

    Type 5: (Greek + Greek)   Compound Terminology

<u>Examples of Latin + Latin Compound Terminology</u>

Latin	Meaning	
norma	rule	
cella	storeroom	
tens	stretch	

Compound Terminology	Meaning	
normocella	normal red cell	
normotensive	normal blood pressure	

Type 2: Examples of Latin + Greek Compound Terminology

Example 1: Norma

Latin	Meaning	Greek	Meaning
norma	normal	blastos	germ
		chroma	color
		glykeros	sweet
		kytos	cell, cyte

Compound Terminology	Meaning
normoblast	normal nucleated red cell
normochromic	a blood cell having normal color
normocyte	normal red blood cell
normoglycemia	normal blood sugar

Example 2: Stomy

Latin	Meaning	
caecus	cecum	
ceco	cecum	
ileum	intestine	
ileo	intestine	

Greek	Meaning	
stoma	mouth	
stomy	opening	

Compound Terminology	Meaning of Compound
cecostomy	surgical opening of cecum
cecoileostomy	connection of cecum and ileum
ileocecostomy	connection of cecum and ileum

Type 3: Example of Latin Modifer + Greek Compound

Latin	English	Meaning	Greek	Meaning
nodus	node	knot	melas	black
nodulus	nodule	small	noma**	spread

Latin *Modifier*	Greek *Compound*	Meaning of Compound
nodular	melanoma	spreading black gangrania
	gangraina	spot

Type 4: Example of Greek Modifer + Latin Compound

Greek	Meaning	Latin	Meaning
dys	bad	ad	attached
hyper	excessive	ren	kidney
hypo	low, small	ia	disease, condition
a	deviation	acidus	sour
		tens	to stretch

Greek Prefix + Latin	Meaning of Compound
anorma*	abnormal, away from normal
dysadrenia	decreased adrenal hormone epinephrine (Greek) or adrenaline (Latin)
hyperacidus	excessive acidity
hypotension	too low blood pressure

Type 5: <u>Examples of Greek + Greek Compound Terminology</u>

Greek	Meaning	Greek	Meaning
lapara	loin	ectomy	cutout
laparo			surgery
nephros	kidney	tomy	surgical incision

Compound Terminology	Meaning	
laparotomy	Incision into the peritoneal cavity	
nephrectomy	Surgical removal of the kidney	

Note:

* "Norma" means "rule" in Latin. Here it is "normal." "Anorma" means "abnormal."

** "Noma" means "spread" in Greek word "nome." (See Type 3)

Greek	Meaning
ana	up (Spelling change: ana — ano) see page 160
op	eye
sia	state of

Compound Terminology	Meaning
anoopsia*, also called hypertropia	eyes deviated upward

Compound Terminology	Meaning	Spelling Changes
thalamos	chamber (a)	thalamus (singular)
		thalami (plural)

(a) Nonmedical meaning of "chamber":

        private room

        bedroom

        meeting room

Medical Compound Terminology (Type 5)

        Hypothalamus

Greek	Meaning	
hypo	below	
thalamos	room (b)	

---

* "Anopsia" means blidness, in which "an" means negative. (see page 168)
   Note that "anoopsia" is different from "anopsia."

(b) The third ventricle of the brain, which relays sensory impluse to the cerebral cortex.

Related Compound Terminology

    Epithalamus: (Upper part including the pineal body)

    Metathalamus: (Medial geniculate body)

    Subthalamus: (Transition zone, for optic impulses)

Table 1: Thesaurus (G) vs (L) related to Blood Circulation

Greek (G) Origin	Latin (L) Origin
Aorta (main trunk)	Venacava (Returning blood main trunk)
Artery (from Arteria in Greek)	Vein (Vescellum means small tubes)
Arterial pressure	Venous pressure
Arteriole	Venule (Small vein), Vebula
Arteriostenosis	Vasoconstriction
Arterio-venous fistula * (G+L)	Venous fistula (connection in Latin)
Angiogensis	Vescellum formation
Artery dilation * (G+L)	Varix (Widening in Latin)
Aortic aneurysm	Varicose aneurysm
Embolism (means plugging)	Infarction (means stuffing)
Thromboangitis (Inflammation)	Phlebitis (Vein inflammation)

* Example of Greek and Latin combination

Dilation is from "dilatere" meaning widening in Latin. In Greek it is called -ectasia or -ectasis.

CHAPTER 3

SPELLING CHANGES

In making compound terminology, prefixes contribute the meaning of the stem word just as an adjective. However, in combined terminology, adjective modifiers further add to the meaning of the compound terminology. (Meanings of "compound" and "combined": see *Chapter 1A & 1B of Part II*)

Some nouns (or stems) become "adjective prefix" by adding "o" at the end. Here, spelling changes for making the prefix are classified into six groups.

Group 1: "al" changes to "o".

Adjectives	Prefixes	Meaning	
abdomin<u>al</u>	abdomin<u>o</u>	abdomen	
bronchi<u>al</u>	bronch<u>o</u>	bronchus	
cerebr<u>al</u>	cerebr<u>o</u>	brain	
crani<u>al</u>	crani<u>o</u>	head bone	
nas<u>al</u>	nas<u>o</u>	nose	
vesic<u>al</u>	vesic<u>o</u>	bladder	

Group 2: "eal" changes to "o".

Adjectives	Prefixes	Meaning	
lact<u>eal</u>	lact<u>o</u>	breast	
mening<u>eal</u>	mening<u>o</u>	membrane in the central nervous system	

Group 3: "um", "a", "e" change to "o".

Nouns	Prefixes or stems	Meaning
cerebr<u>um</u>	cerebr<u>o</u>	brain
stern<u>um</u>	stern<u>o</u>	rib
cardi<u>a</u>	cardi<u>o</u>	heart
stom<u>a</u>	anastom<u>o</u>(sis)	joining vessels
vagin<u>a</u>	vagin<u>o</u>	vagina
ven<u>a</u>	ven<u>o</u>	vein
psych<u>e</u>	psych<u>o</u>	mental faculty

Group 4: "es", "le", "lus" change to "o".

Nouns	Prefixes or stems	Examples
erythrocyt<u>es</u>	erythrocyt<u>o</u>	erythrocyt<u>o</u>sis
thrombocyt<u>es</u>	thrombocyt<u>o</u>	thrombocyt<u>o</u>penia
vesic<u>le</u>	vesic<u>o</u>	vesic<u>o</u>uterine vesic<u>o</u>vaginal
vesic<u>le</u>	vesicul<u>o</u>	vesicul<u>o</u>graphy vesicul<u>o</u>tomy
glomer<u>ulus</u>	glomerul<u>o</u>	glomerul<u>o</u>nephritis

Group 4 Nouns	Meaning		Related Prefixes or Adjectives
erythrocytes	red blood cells		erythr<u>o</u>
thrombosis	clot, thrombus		thromb<u>o</u>
thombocytes	platelet		thomb<u>otic</u>
vesicle	small bladder		cyst<u>o</u>, vesic<u>al</u>
vesicule	blister, seminal vesicle		vesicul<u>ar</u>
glomerulus	small balls in the kidney		glomerul<u>ar</u>

Group 5: Stems plus "i" make adjective of prefixes.

Stem + "i"	Meaning	Examples	
gran<u>i</u>	great	grandiose	
gravi	heavy	gravida	
multi	many	multiple	
novi	new	novitiate	
sani	healthy	sanitation	
testi	witness	testimonial	

Group 6: Stems plus "o" make prefixes.

Stems	Prefixes	Meanings	
angi	angio	vessel	
aux	auxo	grow, multiply	
cardi	cardio	heart	
fiber	fibro	fiber, tissue	
gast	gastro	stomach	
hepat	hepato	liver	
hyster	hystero	uterus	
mast	masto	breast	
metr	metro	uterus	
mamma	mammo	breast	
melan	melano	black	
myel	myelo	marrow	
neur	neuro	nerve	
odont	odonto	teeth	
olig	oligo	few, little	
ovari	ovario	ovary	
path	patho	diseased	
pleur	pleuro	pleural membrane	
proct	procto	rectum, anus	
pseud	pseudo	false	

Stems	Prefixes	Meanings	
splen	spleno	spleen	
spondyl	spondylo	vertebrae	
therm	thermo	heat	
typhl	typhlo	cecum	

CHAPTER 4

GROUPING MEDICAL PREFIXES BY MEANING

1. COLORS

Prefixes	Meanings	Examples	Meaning of Examples
achro	loss of colors	achromatic	
alb	white	albinism	
aniso	dissimilar	anisochromatic	
chloro	green	chloroleukemia	
chro	color	chromatography	
cirrho	yellow	cirrhosis	
cyano	blue	cyanosis	
erythro	red	erythrocyte	
jaune	yellow	jaundice	
leuco	white	leucocyte	
lute	yellow	luteoma	
mel	black	melena	
melano	black	melanonychia	
melano	black	melanosarcoma	
polio	gray	poliosis	

Prefixes	Meanings	Examples	Meaning of Examples
purpur	purple	purpura	
xanth	yellow	xanthodont	

2. LOCATIONS

Prefixes	Meanings	Examples	Meaning of Examples
acro	top, extreme	acrodynia	
ad	attach, near	adherence	
ad	attached	adnexa	
ad	attached	adrenal	
amphi	on both sides	amphicrania	
ante	front	anterior	
antero	front	anteroinferior	
circum	around	circumcision	
dextro	right	dextrocardia	
di	go through	diagonal	
di	opposite	dipolar paranoia	
dorso	back	dorsodynia	
ecto	outside	ectoscopy	
endo	inside	endocrine	
enter	intestine	gastroenteritis	
ento	inside	entoretina	

Prefixes	Meanings	Examples	Meaning of Examples
epi	on, upon	epidermis	
ex	away, out	excrete	
extra	outside	extrauterine	
hemi	half	hemialgia	
infero	below	inferolateral	
inter	between	intercourse	
intra	within	intramuscular	
intra	within	intravenous	
latero	side	lateroabdominal	
medi	middle	medium	
medio	middle	mediodorsal	
meso	middle	mesogastric	
par(a)	beside, around	pararticular	
para	beside, around	paracervical	
peri	around	pericardial	
post	behind	posterior	
retro	behind	retrobulbar	
sub	under	submuscular	
supra	above	supracostal	
trans	across	transfusion	

3. NEGATIVES

Prefixes	Meanings	Examples	Meaning of Examples
a	away	abasia	
a		atrichia	
a	deficiency	avitaminosis	
a		athymia	
a	without	apnea	
a		apepsia	
a		atony	
a	inability	asyndesis	
a		astasia	
a		apraxia	
a		asystole	
a	poor nutrition	atrophy	
a	abnormal	anormal	
ab	remove	abortion	
abs	away from	abstinent	
acy	no	acyesis	
ag	poor growth	agenesis	
am	memory loss	amnesia	
an	loss, without	anhypnia	
an		anorexia	
ana	nothing	anaphia	

Comprehensive Medical Thesaurus

Prefixes	Meanings	Examples	Meaning of Examples
ana	deteriorate	anaplasia	
anen	no brain	anencephaly	
aniso	different, unequal	anisocytosis	
ano	no memory	anomia	
ano	eyesight loss	anopsis	
ano	abnormal shape	anomalous	
anta	against	antagonism	
anti	against	antibiotics	
atelo	incomplete, imperfect	atelocardia	
caco	bad, poor	cacomelia	
cata	down, against	catabiosis	
cata	down	catabolism	
contra	against	contraceptive	
de	decrease	deceleration	
de	oppose, separate	decompose	
de	remove	dehydration	
de	against	detoxication	
dis	against	disinfecting	
dys	difficult, disordered	dyspnea	
hypo	lack of	hypochrosis	
immun	free, safe	immunity	
in	difficult	insomnia	

Prefixes	Meanings	Examples	Meaning of Examples
keno	empty, poor	kenogenesis	
mal	bad, mistake	malodorous	
mal		malpractice	
mal		malaise	
mal	abnormal, bad	malignant	
mal	bad	malnutrition	

4. NUMBERS

Prefixes	Meanings	Examples	Meaning of Examples
bi	two	biennial	
bi	two	bifocal	
cent	hundred	centenary	
dec	ten	decade	
deci	1/10	decigram	
di	twice, apart	division	
diplo	double	diplopia	
duoden	twelve	duodenal	
gem	twin	gemination	
hexa	six	hexahedron	
mono	one, single	monolayer	
octa	eight	octahedron	
qua	four	quarter	

Prefixes	Meanings	Examples	Meaning of Examples
tri	three, triple	triangle	
tetra	four	tetragonal	
uni	one, single	uniformity	

5. QUANTITY

Prefixes	Meanings	Examples	Meaning of Examples
hyper	high, too much	hyperadenoma	
hyper		hyperglycemia	
hypo	little, low	hypochylia	
hypo		hypoemia	
medi	middle	medium	
mio	less, small	miopragia	
multi	many	multigravida	
multi		multipara	
oligo	too little	oligopepsia	
poly	many, much	polyhidrosis	
semi	half, partly	semiconscious	
sub	under	subdermal	
super	too much	superacidity	
ultra	extra	ultrasonic	
ultra		ultraviolet	

6. REGIONS

Prefixes	Meanings	Examples	Meaning of Examples
antero	in front	anterolateral	
dextro	right	dextromanual	
dorso	back, dorsum	dorsoabdominal	
epi	on, upon	epigastric	
latero	side of	lateroabdominal	
levo	left	levoduction	
media	middle	mediastinum	
post	behind	posterior	
sub	under	subcostal	
supra	above	superpubic	
trans	across	transpose	

7. SIZE

Prefixes	Meanings	Examples	Meaning of Examples
auxo	growth	auxocyte	
brachy	short	brachyglossal	
dolich	long	dolichoderas	
giganto	very large	gigantoblast	
giganto	large	gigantocyte	
macro	large	macrophage	
mega	large	megagastria	
micro	small	microbiology	

8. SPEED

Prefixes	Meanings	Examples	Meaning of Examples
brady	slow	bradycardia	
brachy	fast	brachypnea	
de	decrease	decelerate	
tachy	fast	tachycardia	
tachy	fast	tachypnea	

9. TIME SEQUENCE

Prefixes	Meanings	Examples	Meaning of Examples
ante	before	antepyretic	
neo	new	neogenesis	
post	after	postconcussion	
pre	before	premature	
retro	after	retroactive	

CHAPTER 5

Prefixes by Alphabetical Order with Examples
(See Chapter 4 also)

Section A

Prefixes	Meanings	Examples	Meaning of Examples
a	off, without	abacterial	
a		agenesis	
a		aglosia	
a		agnosia	
a		alopecia	
a		aphasia	
a		aplastia	
a		asymmetry	
a		atrophy	
ab	off, without	ablactation	
ab		ablepsia	
abdom	lower part	abdomen	
abdom		abdominal	
abdom		abdominous	
abdomino	abdomen	abdominocentesis	

Comprehensive Medical Thesaurus

Prefixes	Meanings	Examples	Meaning of Examples
abdomino	abdomen	abdominoscope	
achro	loss of color	achromia	
acou	hearing	acoumetry	
acou		acousma	
acro	top, edge	acroesthesia	
acro		acromion	
actino	radiation	actinochemistry	
actino	radiation	actinotherapy	
acu	needle	acuclosure	
acu		acupuncture	
acy	negative	acyesis	
ad	attached	adaptation	
ad		adrenal	
aden	gland	adenalgia	
aden		adenitis	
aden		adenectomy	
adeno	gland	adenoma	
adipo	fat	adipoma	
alb	white	albinism	
alb		albinuria	
albu	white	albumin	
albu		albuminosis	

Prefixes	Meanings	Examples	Meaning of Examples
allo	other	allogamy	
allo		allograft	
alve	cavity	alveolus (dental)	
ambi	both	ambidexterity	
ambi		ambilateral	
amnio	amnion	amniocentesis	
amnio		amnionitis	
amp	both	amphicrania	
amphi	both	amphigenesis	
amphi		amphigenetic	
amphi		amphigonadism	
amphi		amphigony	
ampho	both	amphodiplopia	
amylo	starch	amyloidosis	
amyo	weak muscle	amyocardia	
amyo		amyotaxia	
amyo		amyotonia	
an	no	anosmia	
ana	no feeling	analgesia	
ana		analgesic	
ana		anaphia	
andro	masculine	androgen	

Prefixes	Meanings	Examples	Meaning of Examples
andro	masculine	andromania	
ane	no feeling	anesthesia	
ane	lack of	anemia	
ane		anemic	
angi	blood vessel	angina pectoris	
angi		angiitis	
angio	blood vessel	angiocolitis	
angio		angiography	
angio		angioma	
angio		angioplasty	
aniso	dissimilar	anisochromatic	
aniso		anisocytosis	
aniso	dissimilar	anisodont	
ankyl	stiffening	ankylo	
ankyl		ankylodactylia	
ankyl		ankylosis	
ano	no memory	anomia	
ano	lack of	anopia	
anod	no pain	anodinia	
anod		anodinous	
anod		anodynia	
anor	no (appetite)	anorexia	

Prefixes	Meanings	Examples	Meaning of Examples
anor	abnormal (eye sight)	anorthopia	
anos	anus	anoscope	
anos		anosigmodoscopy	
anox	lack of oxygen	anoxia	
ante	front	antecubital	
ante	before	antefebrile	
antero	front	anteroposterior	
anti	against, stop	antibacterial	
anti		antibromic	
anti		anticoagulant	
anti		antidiarrheal	
anti		antidote	
anti		antiemetic	
anti		antilethargic	
anti		antineuralgic	
anti		antiparasitic	
anti		antiphthisic	
anti		antipruritic	
anti		antipyretic	
anti		antisepsis	
anti		antiseptic	
anti		antiserum	

Comprehensive Medical Thesaurus

Prefixes	Meanings	Examples	Meaning of Examples
anti	against, stop	antithyroid	
anti	against, stop	antitoxin	
anti		antitubercular	
aort	main aorta	aortitis	
aort	blood trunk	aortography	
apo	derivation	aponeurosis	
apo		apophysis	
apo		apoprotein	
arch(e)	first, main	archespore	
arterio	blood trunk	arteriosclerosis	
arthr	joint	arthralgia	
arthr		arthritis	
arthr		arthroscopy	
articul	joint	articulation	
atax	disorder	ataxia	
atax		ataxic	
atel	poor health	atelectasis	
atelo	imperfect	atelocardia	
atelo	poor growth	atelorrachidia	
athero	cholesterol, lipids	atherosclerosis	
athero	mass of fat	atheromatosis	
atre	close	atresia	

Prefixes	Meanings	Examples	Meaning of Examples
atreto	no opening	atretorrhinia	
audi	to hear	audiometry	
auto	own self	autoimmunity	
auto		autonomic	
auxe	growth	auxesis	
auxo	growth	auxospore	
ax	axis	axial	
azo	containing nitrogen	azotemia	
azoo	without	azoospermia	

Prefixes	Meanings	Examples	Meaning of Examples

Section B

Prefixes	Meanings	Examples	Meaning of Examples
bacil	bacterium	bacillicide	
bacil		bacillus	
bacter		bacteriology	
balano	penis	balanoplasty	
bary	difficult	barycoia	
basal	fundamental	basal cell	
basila	base	basila artery	
basilo		basiloma	
baso	basic	basophil	
bili	bile	biliation	
biliary	bile	biliary duct	
bio	life	biogenesis	
bio		biofeedback	
bio		bioscopy	
blast	embryonic	blastoma	
blenn	flow of mucus	blennostasis	
blenn		blennuria	
blephar	eyelids	blepharitis	
blepharo		blepharochalasis	
blepharo		blepharoplasty	
botulism	food poisoning	botulismtoxin	

Prefixes	Meanings	Examples	Meaning of Examples
brachi	arm	brachialgia	
brachy	short	brachymetropia	
brachy	fast	brachypnea	
brady	slow	bradycardia	
brady		bradykinesia	
brady		bradyglossia	
bronchi	bronchus	bronchial	
bronchi		bronchitis	
brancho		branchoscopy	
burs	bursa	bursitis	

Section C

Prefixes	Meanings	Examples	Meaning of Examples
caco	bad, ill, poor	cacochylia	
caco		cacoepy	
caco		cacopathy	
caco		cacosmia	
calor	heat	calorie	
canal	small tube	canaliculus	
cancer	malignant tumor	cancerous	
carcin	cancer	carcinogen	
carcin	cancer	carcinoma	
carcin		carcinectomy	
cardi	heart	cardiectomy	
cardi		cardiac arrest	
cardio	heart	cardiogram	
cardio		cardiomyopathy	
cardio		cardiopulmonary	
cardio		cardiovascular	
carpal	wrist	carpal tunnel syndrome	
carpo	wrist	carpopedal spasm	
cata	down, under	catabolism	
catal	hardening	catalepsy	
cav	hallow	cavity	

Prefixes	Meanings	Examples	Meaning of Examples
ceco	cecum	cecostomy	
ceco		cecoptosis	
celia	abdomen	celia block	
celio	abdomen	celioma	
cell	cellular	cellulitis	
cell	tissue unit	cellular	
ceno	empty (keno)	cenosis	
ceno	new	cenogenesis	
centro	center	centrosome	
cephalo	head	cephalocele	
cerebell	small brain	cerebellum	
cerebra	cerebrum (big brain)	cerebra thrombosis	
cerebro		cerebrospinal	
cervic	neck	cervical cap	
cervico	neck	cervicodynia	
cheil	lip	cheilitis	
cheil		cheiloplasty	
chemo	chemical	chemoprophylaxis	
chemo		chemotherapy	
chiro	hand	chiromania	
chiro		chiropractor	
chloro	green	chlorophyl	

Comprehensive Medical Thesaurus

Prefixes	Meanings	Examples	Meaning of Examples
cholangi	bile duct	cholangitis	
cholangio	bile duct	cholangioma	
cholangia		cholangiogram	
chole	bile	cholelith	
cholecyst	gallbladder	cholecystectomy	
chondro	cartilage	chondroarthritis	
chondro		chondrocarcinoma	
chondro		chondromatosis	
chorio	fetal membrane	chorioangioma	
chorio		choriocarcinoma	
chorion	fetal membrane	chorionitis	
chorioretino	retina membrane	chorioretinopathyy	
chro	color	chromasia	
chromo	color	chromometer	
chyl	cloudy liquid	chylous	
cili	eyelid	ciliary	
col	colon	colectomy	
col		colonoscopy	
colp	vagina	colpalgia	
colpo		colpocystitis	
colpo		colpopathy	
colpo		colposcope	

Prefixes	Meanings	Examples	Meaning of Examples
cost	rib	costalgia	
costo	rib	costotomy	
crani	skull	cranium	
cranio	skull	craniotomy	
crypto	hidden	cryptococcosis	
crypto		cryptomenorrhea	
cyst	bladder, pouch	cystectomy	
cysto	bladder	cystodynia	
cysto		cystoscopy	
cyto	cell	cytology	
cyto		cytoma	
cyto		cytochemistry	
cyto		cytodieresis	
cyto		cytogenesis	
cyto	cell	cytokinesis	

Section D

Prefixes	Meanings	Examples	Meaning of Examples
de	decrease	decelerate	
de	remove	deodorant	
de	decrease	dementia	
dec	ten	decade	
deci	1/10	decigram	
dent	teeth, tooth	denture	
derma	skin	dermatitis	
dermo	skin	dermotheraphy	
desicc	dry	desiccant	
desmo	ligament	desmocytoma	
desmo		desmosis	
dextro	right	dextrocerebral	
dia	apart, diffraction	dialysis	
dicho	into two	dichotomy	
didym	testicle	didymalgia	
didym		didymitis	
digit	finger	digital prostate exam	
dipl	double	diplopia	
diplo	double	diplococcus	
dorso	back	dorsodynia	
duode	twelve	duodenitis	

Prefixes	Meanings	Examples	Meaning of Examples
duodeno	duodenum	duodenography	
dys	bad, disorder	dysacusia	
dys		dyslexia	
dys		dysmenorrhea	
dys	pain	dyspareunia	
dys	bad, disorder	dyspepsia	
dys		dysphasia	
dys		dysphonia	
dys		dyspnea	
dys		dystocia	
dys		dystonia	
dys		dystrophy	
dys		dysuria	

Prefixes	Meanings	Examples	Meaning of Examples

Section E

Prefixes	Meanings	Examples	Meaning of Examples
echo	sound	echocardiography	
ect	outside, outward	ectal	
ecto	outside	ectoblast	
ecto		ectopic pregnancy	
em	in	embolism	
em	on	embrocation	
embol	plug	embolectomy	
embryo	baby	embryology	
encephal	brain	encephalitis	
encephal		encephalomeningitis	
encephal		encephalopathy	
encephal		encephalospinal	
end	inside	endangiitis	
end		endaortitis	
end		endarteritis	
end		endarterectomy	
endo	inside	endocarditis	
endo		endocrine	
endo	nerve	endodontitis	
endo	inside	endogenous	
endo		endometritis	

Prefixes	Meanings	Examples	Meaning of Examples
endo	inside	endoscope	
endo		endosteum	
ent	inside	entoptic	
ent		entotic	
enter	intestine	enteritis	
entero	intestine	enteroanastomosis	
entero		enterocele	
entero		enterocolitis	
entero		enterogastritis	
entero		enterohemorrhage	
entero	intestine	enteroparalysis	
entero		enterotomy	
entero		enterotoxin	
entero		enteroscope	
entero		enterostenosis	
entero		enterostomy	
entero		enterotomy	
ento	inside	entocele	
ento		entogastric	
ento		entorrhagia	
epi	on	epicardium	
epi		epicranium	

Comprehensive Medical Thesaurus

Prefixes	Meanings	Examples	Meaning of Examples
epi	spread over	epidemic	
epi	skin	epidermal	
epi	attached to	epididymis	
epi	on	epiglottiditis	
epi		epiglottis	
episio	pubic region	episiocele	
episio		episiotomy	
epithel	covering skin	epithelia	
epithel		epithelioma	
eroto	sexual	erotomania	
eroto		erotophobia	
eryth	red	erythema	
erythro	red	erythroblast	
erythro	red	erythrocyte	
erythro		erythrocytosis	
erythro		erythroleukemia	
erythro		erythropoiesis	
erythro		erythropoietin	
eso	within	esophagitis	
eso		esophagus	
esthe	feeling	esthesia	
etio	cause	etiology	

Prefixes	Meanings	Examples	Meaning of Examples
eu	good, well	eucholia	
eu		eupepsia	
eury	broad, wide	eurythermal	
ex	outside, eliminate	excision	
ex	away, outside	excrement	
ex	outside, outward	exodontia	
ex		exhale	
ex		exophthalmia	
ex		exostosis	
exo	outside, outward	exocrine	
exo		exoderm	
exo		exothermic	
exo		exotoxin	
exo		exotropia	
extra	beyond, outside	extracapsular	
extra		extracellular	
extra		extracoronal	
extra		extracostal	
extra		extradural	
extra		extraocular	
extra		extravasation	
extra		extravascular	

Section F

Prefixes	Meanings	Examples	Meaning of Examples
facio	face	facioplegia	
facio		facioplasty	
fasci	fibrous tissue	fascia	
fasci		fascioplasty	
fasci		fasciotomy	
febri	fever	febrile	
femoral	thigh	femoral artery	
feti	fetus	feticide	
feti	sex	fetish	
feto	fetus	fetoscope	
fibro	fiber	fibroadenoma	
fibro		fibrocarcinoma	
fibro		fibrochondroma	
fibro		fibromyositis	
fibro		fibroneuroma	
fibro		fibrosarcoma	
fila	thread	filaceous	
fiss	cleft, groove, split	fissure	
for	opening	foramen	
fore	before, front	forebrain	
fore		foregut	

Prefixes	Meanings	Examples	Meaning of Examples
fore	before, front	forehead	
fore		foreplay	
fore		foreskin	
front	front	frontal vein	

Section G

Prefixes	Meanings	Examples	Meaning of Examples
galacto	milk	galactorrhea	
galacto		galactosemia	
galacto		galactotherapy	
gam	join, unite	gamete	
gameto	reproductive cell	gametogenesis	
gamo	union	gamophobia	
gangli	ganglion	ganglion	
gangli		ganglionic blockade	
gangli		ganglionitis	
gastr	stomach	gastrinoma	
gastri	stomach	gastritis	
gastro	stomach	gastroblennorrhea	
gastro		gastrocolitis	
gastro		gastroduodenal	
gastro		gastroenteritis	
gastro		gastroesophageal	
gastro		gastrostomy	
gastro		gastronephritis	
gelat	freeze	gelation	
gelat		gelattinous	
gen	produce	generate	

Prefixes	Meanings	Examples	Meaning of Examples
gen	produce	genesis	
gen		genital	
gene	origin	genetic	
genito	genital	genitourinary	
geo	earth, soil	geofiology	
geo		geotrickosis	
geria	old age	geriatrics	
gerio	old age	geriopsychosis	
geron	old age	gerontology	
germ	sprout	germicide	
germ		germinate	
gesta	develop fetus	gestation	
gingi	gingiva	gingivitis	
glia	gluey	glia cell	
glio	neuroglia	glioblastoma	
glio		gliosarcoma	
glio		gliosis	
gloss	tongue	glossalgia	
gloss		glossopharyngeal	
glott	tongue	glottitis	
glu	glucagon	glucagon hormone	
gluco	sugar, sweet	glucosuria	

Prefixes	Meanings	Examples	Meaning of Examples
glyco	sweetness,	glycogen	
glyco		glycopolyuria	
glyco		glycorrhea	
glyco		glycosuria	
gnath	jaw	gnathodynia	
gnath		gnathoplasty	
gonad	seed producing	gonadal	
gonad		gonadopathy	
gonad		gonadotherapy	
gonio	angle	goniometer	
gonio		gonioscope	
gono	semen, seed	gonococcus	
gono		gonocyte	
gono		gonorrhea	
gony	knee	gonycampsis	
gony		gonyoncus	
gyne	female	gynecology	

Section H

Prefixes	Meanings	Examples	Meaning of Examples
hem	blood	hemangioma	
hemart	fault (in Greek)	hemartoma	
hemat	blood	hematemesis	
hemat		hematuria	
hemato	blood	hematocele	
hemato		hematochezia	
hemato		hematologist	
hemato		hematoma	
hemi	half	hemialgia	
hemi		hemianopsia	
hemi		hemicrania	
hemi		hemifacial	
hemi		hemiplegia	
hemo	blood	hemochromatosis	
hemo		hemoconcentration	
hemo		hemodialysis	
hemo		hemofiltration	
hemo		hemoglobin	
hemo		hemolysis	
hemo		hemolytic anemia	
hemo		hemoperfusion	

Comprehensive Medical Thesaurus

Prefixes	Meanings	Examples	Meaning of Examples
hemo	bleeding	hemophilia	
hemo		hemoptysis	
hemo		hemorrhage	
hemo		hemorrhoid	
hemo		hemosiderosis	
hemo		hemostasis	
hemo		hemostatic	
hemo		hemothorax	
hepat	liver	hepatitis	
hepat		hepatoma	
hernia	rupture	herniorrhaphy	
hernio		herniotomy	
herp	creep	herpangina	
herp		herpetic	
hetero	another, different	heterochromatin	
hetero		heterochromosome	
hetero		heterogamy	
hetero		heterogenesis	
hetero		heterogeneity	
hetero		heterosexual	
hetero		heterotropia	
hidro	sweat	hidrodermia	

Prefixes	Meanings	Examples	Meaning of Examples
histo	tissue structure	histocyte	
histo		histocompatiblity	
histo		histology	
histo		histoplasma	
homeo	similar	homeopathy	
homeo		homeostasis	
homo	same	homogeneity	
homo		homogenization	
homo		homosexual	
horm	stimulate for goal	hormism	
hormon	to begin action	hormonogenic	
hydro	water	hydrocele	
hydro		hydrocephalus	
hydro		hydroma	
hydro		hydronephrosis	
hydro		hydrosalpinx	
hyper	super	hyperglycemia	
hyper		hypertension	
hyper		hyperthyroidism	
hyper		hypertrophic	
hypno	sleep	hypnopathy	
hypno		hypnosis	

Comprehensive Medical Thesaurus

Prefixes	Meanings	Examples	Meaning of Examples
hypno	sleep	hypnotic	
hypo	poor health	hypochondria	
hypo		hypochylia	
hypo	below	hypodermic	
hypo	low	hypoglycemia	
hypo		hyponatremia	
hypo		hypophysis	
hypo		hypoplasia	
hypo		hypothalamic	
hypo		hypothyroidism	
hypo		hypoxemia	
hyster	uterus	hysteralgia	
hyster		hysterectomy	
hystero		hysterocele	
hystero		hysterodynia	
hystero		hysteromyoma	
hystero		hysteromyotomy	
hystero		hysterorrhexis	
hystero		hysterospasm	
hystero		hysterotomy	

Section I

Prefixes	Meanings	Examples	Meaning of Examples
iatro	medical	iatrogenic	
icter	jaundice	icterus	
idio	own, peculiar	idiopathic	
idio	retarded	idiot	
idio	own, peculiar	idiotropic	
ileo	ileum	ileotomy	
ileo		ileostomy	
immune	free, safe	immunization	
immune		immunize	
immune		immunogen	
immune		immunotoxin	
infra	below	infra-axillary	
infra		infracostal	
infra		infrared	
infuse	penetrate	infusible	
infuse		infusion	
inter	between	interaction	
inter		interarticular	
inter		interbreeding	
inter		intercalation	
inter		intercellular	

Prefixes	Meanings	Examples	Meaning of Examples
inter	between	intercourse	
inter		intermittent	
intra	inside	intracranial	
intra		intradermal	
intra		intra-abdominal	
intra		intranasal	
intra		intravenous	
intro	inside	introitus	
intu	insert, into	intubate	
ipsi/ipso	same side	ipsilateral	
irido	iris, rainbow	iridotomy	
iso	equal, or related	isoenzyme	
iso		isotope	
iso		isotropic	
iso		isogamy	

Section J

Prefixes	Meanings	Examples	Meaning of Examples
jejuno	jejunum	jejunal	
jejuno		jejunectomy	
jejuno		jejunocolostomy	
jug	yoke	conjugal	
jug		jugal	
jugu	neck, throat	jugular	
jugu		jugulum	
juxta	beside, near	juxtapose	
juxta		juxtaspinal	
juxta		juxtaepiphysial	
juxta		juxtaposition	
juxta		juxtaarticular	

Section K

Prefixes	Meanings	Examples	Meaning of Examples
karyo	nucleus, cytology	karyology	
karyo	nucleus	karyolysis	
kel	tumor	keloma	
kel		keloid	
keno	empty	kenophobia	
kera	horn	keratoma	
kera		keratitis	
kera		keratosis	
kera		keratotomy	
kypho	hump	kyphoscoliosis	
kypho		kyphosis	

Section L

Prefixes	Meanings	Examples	Meaning of Examples
labio	lips	labionasal	
labio		labiolingual	
lacri	tear	lacrimation	
lact	milk	lactalbumin	
lact		lactate	
lact		lactoscope	
lact		lactogen	
lact		lactose	
lact		lactosuria	
lact		lactovegetation	
lalio	talk	laliophobia	
lalo	talk	lalopathy	
lamin	layer	laminar	
lamin	layer	laminectomy	
laparo	flank	laparoscope	
laparo		laparotomy	
laryng	larynx	laryngitis	
laryng		laryngectomy	
laryng		laryngocele	
latero	side	laterodeviation	
leio	smooth	leiomyoma	

Prefixes	Meanings	Examples	Meaning of Examples
lepto	thin	leptodermic	
lepto		leptomeningitis	
leuco	white	leucocyte	
leuco		leucoderma	
leuco		leucopenia	
lipo	fat	lipoblast	
lipo		lipochondroma	
lipo		lipogenic	
lipo		lipoma	
lipo		lipomyoma	
lipo		lipoprotein	
lipo		liposarcoma	
lipo		liposuction	
litho	calculus, stone	lithogenesis	
litho		lithotomy	
litho		lithotripsy	
lymph	clear body fluid	lymphocyte	
lymph		lymphosarcoma	
lymph		lymphadenoma	

Section M

Prefixes	Meanings	Examples	Meaning of Examples
macro	large	macrophage	
mal	abnormal, ill	malalignment	
mal		malformation	
mal		malignant	
mal		malingerer	
mal		malnutrition	
mal		malpractice	
mamm	breast	mammalgia	
mamm		mammograph	
mamm		mammoplasty	
mast	breast	mastalgia	
mast		mastectomy	
mast		mastitis	
mast		mastoid	
mast		mastopathy	
mega	great	megacolon	
megalo	great	megalomania	
meio	becoming smaller	meiosis	
mel	black	melena	
melan	black	melanocyte	
melan		melanoma	

Comprehensive Medical Thesaurus

Prefixes	Meanings	Examples	Meaning of Examples
mening	brain membrane or spinal cord membrane	meningitis	
meningo		meningocele	
meningo		meningococcus	
meningo		meningopathy	
meno	menses	menopause	
meno		menorrhea	
mer	part, portion	meropia	
mer	lacking	merosmia	
mero	part	meroblast	
mero		merogenesis	
mesen	middle	mesencephalon	
mesen		mesentery	
meso	middle, membrane	mesocolon	
meso		mesogastric	
meso		mesogastrium	
meta	change, exchange	metabolism	
meta		metachromasia	
meta		metagenesis	
meta		metamorphosis	
meta		metaplasia	
meta		metastasis	
metr	uterus	metralgia	

Prefixes	Meanings	Examples	Meaning of Examples
metr	uterus	metratrophia	
metr		metrectasis	
metr		metrectomy	
metr		metremia	
metro	uterus	metrodynia	
micro	small	microbe	
micro		microbiologist	
mio	becoming less	miopragia	
mio		miosis	
mito	threadlike	mitochondria	
mito		mitogenesis	
mito		mitosis	
mono	one, single	monoblast	
mono		monocyte	
morph	form, shape	morphea	
morpho	form, shape	morphogenesis	
morpho		morphogeny	
morpho		morphology	
muco	mucus, mucous	mucocele	
muco		mucosa	
multi	many	multicellular	
multi		multigravida	

Prefixes	Meanings	Examples	Meaning of Examples
muta	change	mutation	
my	muscle	myasthenia	
myce	fungus	mycetoma	
myco	fungus	mycobacterium complex	
myco		mycology	
myco		mycoplasma	
myco		mycosis	
myelo	marrow	myelocele	
myelo		myelocyte	
myelo		myeloma	
myelo		myelopathy	
myelo		myelotomy	
myo	muscle	myocarditis	
myo		myoclonus	
myo		myopathy	
myo		myositis	
myxo	mucus	myxofibroma	
myxo		myxoma	
myxo		myxosarcoma	
myxo		myxovirus	

Section N

Prefixes	Meanings	Examples	Meaning of Examples
narco	stupor, lethargy	narcolepsy	
narco		narcosis	
narco		narcotic	
nas	nasal	nasalis	
naso		nasogastric (intubation)	
naso		nasolacrimal	
naso		nasopharyngeal	
necro	death	necrobiosis	
necro		necropsy	
nemato	threadlike	nematode	
nemato		nematosis	
neo	new	neoblastic	
neo		neogenesis	
neo		neonatology	
neo		neoplasia	
neo		neoplasm	
nephr	nephros (kidney)	nephrectomy	
nephr		nephritis	
nephr		nephrocalcinosis	
nephr		nephropathy	
nephr		nephrosclerosis	

Comprehensive Medical Thesaurus

Prefixes	Meanings	Examples	Meaning of Examples
nephr	kidney	nephrostomy	
nephr		nephrotomy	
neur	nerves	neuralgia	
neur		neurasthenia	
neur		neuritis	
neuro		neuroarthropathy	
neuro	nerves	neuroblastoma	
neuro		neurocanal	
neuro		neurocardiac	
neuro		neurocytoma	
neuro		neurodermatitis	
neuro		neurodynia	
neuro		neurogenic	
neuro		neurohormonal	
neuro		neuroma	
neuro		neuropathy	
neuro		neurosarcoma	
neuro		neurosis	
neuro		neurospasm	
neuro		neurotic	
noct	night	nocturia	
noct		nocturnal	

212

Prefixes	Meanings	Examples	Meaning of Examples
nod	knot	nodule	
noso	disease	nosocomial infection	
noso		nosology	
nota	back	notalgia	
nutri	nourishment	nutrition	
nyct	night	nyctophobia	
nymph	labia minora	nymphitis	
nymph	labia minora	nymphotomy	

Section O

Prefixes	Meanings	Examples	Meaning of Examples
odont	tooth or teeth	odontectomy	
odont		odontitis	
odont		odontobothritis	
odont		odontogenesis	
odont		odontoma	
odont		odontoneuralgia	
odyno	pain	odynophagia	
olig	few, little	oligemia	
olig		oligomenorrhea	
olig		oligospermia	
olig		oliguria	
omo	shoulder	omodynia	
omphal	umbilicus	omphallocele	
omphal		omphaloma	
onco	swelling tumor	oncocyte	
onco		oncology	
onycho	nail	onycholysis	
onycho		onychoma	
oophoro	ovary	oophoroma	
ophthalm	eye	ophthalmia	
orchi	testis	orchialgia	

Prefixes	Meanings	Examples	Meaning of Examples
orchi		orchitis	
orchi	testis	orchiectomy	
ortho	normal	orthodromic	
ortho	correct, normal	orthopedist	
ortho		orthodontist	
osmi	odor	osmia	
osmi		osmidrosis	
osmi		osmidrosis axillae	
osmo	odors	osmolagnia	
osmo	osmosis, impulse	osmotic pressure	
oss	bone	osseous	
oss		ossicle	
oss		ossify	
osteo	bone	osteomyelitis	
osteo		osteonecrosis	
oto	ear	otodynia	
oto		otoneuralgia	
oto		otorrhea	
oto		otoscopy	
ovari	ovary	ovariocentesis	
ovi	egg	oviduct	
ovo	egg	ovoblast	

Comprehensive Medical Thesaurus

Prefixes	Meanings	Examples	Meaning of Examples
ovo		ovoid	
oxi	oxygen	oxidizer	
oxy	oxygen, sour	oxydase	
oxy		oxyhemoglobin	
oxy	acid	oxyntic	

Prefixes	Meanings	Examples	Meaning of Examples

Section P

Prefixes	Meanings	Examples	Meaning of Examples
palat	palate	palatine bone	
palm	palm	palmaris	
pan	all	pandemic	
papilla	nipple	papillitis	
papilla		papilloma	
papillo		papillotomy	
para	beside, similar	para-articular	
para		parabiotic	
para		paracentesis	
para		paraganglion	
para	beside, around	paracervical block	
para	beside, disorder	parahepatitis	
para		parainfection	
para		paranomia	
para		paranoia, paranoid	
para		paraphilia	
para		paraplegia	
patho	disease	pathogenesis	
patho		pathology	
patho		pathophysiology	
pecto	chest	pectoralis	

Comprehensive Medical Thesaurus

Prefixes	Meanings	Examples	Meaning of Examples
pediatric	child	pediatrician	
pedo	child	pedodontics	
peps	digestion	pepsin	
per	through	percutaneous	
peri	around	perianal	
peri		periarteritis	
peri		pericardial	
peri		pericarditis	
peri		pericardium	
peri		periproctal	
peri		peritonitis	
pero	deformed, congenital	peromelia	
pero		peronia	
petr	stone	petrification	
petr		petrify	
phaco	lens	phacomalacia	
phaco		phacosclerosis	
phago	eating	phagocyte	
phago		phagocytosis	
phall	penis	phallalgia	
phall		phallus	
pharyng	throat	pharyngectomy	

218

Prefixes	Meanings	Examples	Meaning of Examples
pharyng	throat	pharyngitis	
phleb	vein	phlebectomy	
phleb		phlebitis	
phlebo	vein	phlebothrombosis	
phren	diaphragm	phrenospasm	
phyl	guard	phylaxis	
plasma	blood, liquid	plasmacytoma	
plasma		plasmapheresis	
platy	broad, flat	platypodia	
pleur	rib, pleura	pleuralgia	
pleur		pleurisy	
pleuro		pleurocentesis	
pleuro		pleurodynia	
pleuro		pleurotomy	
plex	strike, stroke	plexor	
plex	network	plexus	
plic	fold, ridge	plica	
pneu	air, gas	pneumatocele	
pneu		pneumectomy	
pneumo	lung	pneumococcus	
pneumo		pneumoconiosis	
pneumo		pneumonia	

Comprehensive Medical Thesaurus

Prefixes	Meanings	Examples	Meaning of Examples
pneumo	lung	pneumonitis	
pneumo		pneumonotomy	
pneumo		pneumosilicosis	
pneumo		pneumothorax	
poie	formation, production	poiesis	
poikilo	irregular, varied	poikilocytosis	
poikilo		poikiloderma	
polio	gray	polioencephalitis	
polio		polioencephalomyelitis	
polio		poliomyelitis	
poly	many	polyarthritis	
poly		polychromatic	
poly		polydipsia	
poly		polymyalgia	
poly		polyuria	
post	after	postmortem	
post	behind	posterior	
pre	before	precancerous	
pre		precocious	
pre		precordial	
pre		precursor	
pre		premenstrual	

220

Prefixes	Meanings	Examples	Meaning of Examples
pre		prepuce	
presby	old man, senior	presbyatriys	
presby		presbycardia	
presby		presbycusis	
presby		presbyopia	
prim	first	primary	
prim		primigravida	
prim		primipara	
prim		primordial	
pro	ahead	prognosis	
proct	rectum	proctalgia	
proct		proctitis	
proct		proctectomy	
proct		proctocele	
proct		proctologist	
proct		proctoscope	
pros	look, forward	prospective	
prosta	prostate	prostatitis	
prostho	addition	prosthodontia	
proteo	protein	proteolysis	
proteo		proteolytic	
proto	first	protopathy	

Prefixes	Meanings	Examples	Meaning of Examples
pseudo	false	pseudogout	
pseudo		pseudopregnancy	
psor	itching	psoriasis	
psor		psoriatic (arthritis)	
psych	mind	psychedelic	
psych		psychiatric	
psycho	mind	psychoanalysis	
psycho		psychology	
psycho		psychoneurosis	
psycho		psychopath	
psycho		psychopathology	
psycho		psychosis	
psycho		psychotherapy	
pueri	child	puericulture	
pulmon	lung	pulmonary edema	
pulmon		pulmonary embolism	
pulmon		pulmonary emphysema	
pulmon		pulmonary stenosis	
pulmon		pulmonectomy	
pulmon		pulmonic	
punct	point	punctum lacrimale	
punct		puncture	

Prefixes	Meanings	Examples	Meaning of Examples
pyelo	kidney	pyelography	
pyelo		pyelonephritis	
pyo	pus	pyocenosis	
pyo		pyoderma	
pyo		pyogenic	
pyo		pyosis	
pyreto	fever	pyretotherapy	
pyro	fire, heat	pyromania	
pyro		pyrophobia	
pyro		pyrosis	

Section Q

Prefixes	Meanings	Examples	Meaning of Examples
quadr	four	quadriplegia	
quin	fifth	quintana fever	
quin		quintuplet	

Section R

Prefixes	Meanings	Examples	Meaning of Examples
rachio	spine	rachiodynia	
rachio		rachiopathy	
radio	radiation	radioactive	
radio		radiology	
radio		radiotherapy	
ren	kidney	renal angiography	
ren		renal biopsy	
reticul	netlike	reticular	
reticul		reticulocyte	
retina	netlike nerve tissue	retina	
retina		retinitis	
retino		retinopathy	
retro	backward, behind	retroclusion	
retro		retroflexion	
retro		retrograde	
retro		retrogression	
rheo	current, flow	rheometer	
rheumat	inflammatory	rheumatic fever	
rhin	nose	rhinitis	
rhino	nose	rhinoantritis	
rhino		rhinocleisis	

Prefixes	Meanings	Examples	Meaning of Examples
rhino	nose	rhinolalia	
rhino		rhinolaryngitis	
rhino		rhinoplasty	
rhino		rhinorrhea	
rhino	nose	rhinoscope	
rhytid	wrinkle	rhytidectomy	
rhytid		rhytidoplasty	
rhizo	spinal root	rhizotomy	

Section S

Prefixes	Meanings	Examples	Meaning of Examples
saccade	jerky	saccadic movement	
saccharo	sugar	saccharogen	
saccharo		saccharosuria	
sacro	sacrum	sacroiliac	
sarcro		sarcrospinal	
salic	salicin acid	salicylate	
salic		salicylic acid	
salping	tube, fallopian tube, salpinx	salpingitis	
salpingo		salpingostomy	
san	healthy	sane	
san		sanity	
sanita	health	sanitarium	
sanita		sanitation	
sapo	soap	saponin	
sapro	decay	saprogenic	
sapro		saprophyte	
sarco	flesh	sarcoidosis	
sarco		sarcoma	
scab	dry skin, eschar	scabicide	
schisto	cleft, split	schistocyte	
schizo	division, split	schizocyte	

Prefixes	Meanings	Examples	Meaning of Examples
schizo	split	schizophrenia	
scirrho	hard cancer	scirrhous carinoma	
scler	hard	scleriasis	
scler		scleritis	
sclera	hard	sclera	
sclero	hard	sclerosis	
sclero		sclerocataract	
sclero		scleroderma	
scolio	crooked, twisted	scoliosis	
scoto	darkness	scotoma	
semi	half	semicoma	
semi		semilunar valve	
sero	serum	serology	
sialo	saliva	sialoadenitis	
sialo		sialorrhea	
sidero	iron	siderosis	
sito	food	sitology	
sito		sitophobia	
soma	body	somatic	
sphygmo	pulse	sphygmomanometer	
spino	spine	spinocerebellar	
splanchno	internal organ	splanchnocele	

Comprehensive Medical Thesaurus

Prefixes	Meanings	Examples	Meaning of Examples
splanchno	internal organ	splanchnodynia	
splen	spleen	splenectomy	
spleno	spleen	splenocele	
spleno		splenomegaly	
spondyl	vertebra	spondylarthritis	
spondyl		spondylodynia	
spondyl		spondylopathy	
spondyl		spondylosis	
spondyl		spondylitis	
spongio	resilient	spongioblastoma	
steato	fat	steatolysis	
steato		steatoma	
steato		steatorrhea	
stell	star shape	stellate fracture	
steno	narrow	stenosis	
stereo	solid	stereoarthrolysis	
stereo	three-dimensional	stereoscopy	
stetho	chest	stethoscope	
sterno	sternum	sternoclavicular	
sterno		sternocostal	
sterno		sternotomy	
stomato	mouth	stomatotitis	

Prefixes	Meanings	Examples	Meaning of Examples
stomato	mouth	stomatotody-sosmia	
stomato		stomatotosis	
strepto	twisted	streptococcus	
sub	near, under	subabdominal	
sub		subacute	
sub		subconscious	
sub		subcutaneous	
sub		subdermal	
sub		subdermal	
sub		subglossal	
sub		substernal (goiter)	
sub		subungual (hematoma)	
succ	juice	succinic acid	
succ		succus	
sudo	sweat	sudoriferous gland	
sudo		sudorrhea	
super	excess	superinfection	
super		supersensitive	
sym	union	symbiosis	
sym		symbiotic	
sym		sympathetic	
sym		symphysis	

Prefixes	Meanings	Examples	Meaning of Examples
syn	union	synapse	
syn		synaptic	
syn		synergic	
syn		synthesize	

Section T

Prefixes	Meanings	Examples	Meaning of Examples
tabe	wasting	tabesdorsalis	
tachy	rapid	tachycardia	
tachy		tachyphagia	
tachy		tachyrhythmia	
tact	touch	tactile	
tars	edge of foot or eyelid	tarsitis	
tars		tarsus	
tarso		tarsoplasty	
tarso		tarsorrhaphy	
tarso		tarsotomy	
tax	order of division or arrangement	taxology	
tax		taxonomy	
teg	cover	tegmen	
teg		tegment	
tela	web	telalgia	
tela		telangioma	
tela		telangiitis	
tele	end	telecepter	
tele	far away	telepathy	
tele		teletherapy	
telo	end	teloblast	

Comprehensive Medical Thesaurus

Prefixes	Meanings	Examples	Meaning of Examples
telo	end	telophase	
ten	tendon	tenorrhaphy	
ten		tenosynovitis	
terato	monster	teratoblastoma	
terato		teratogenesis	
terato		teratoma	
tetan	tetanus	tetanoid	
tetan		tetanus	
tetra	four	tetragon	
tetra		tetrapod	
thel	nipple	thelarche	
thel		theleplasty	
thel		thelitis	
therm	heat	thermocautery	
therm		thermofuge	
therm		thermotherapy	
thio	sulfur	thiocyanate	
thoraco	chest	thoracoabdominal	
thoraco		thoracocentesis	
thoraco		thoracodorsal	
thoraco		thoracotomy	
thrombo	clot	thromboangiitis	

Prefixes	Meanings	Examples	Meaning of Examples
thrombo	clot	thrombocytosis	
thrombo		thrombosis	
thym	strong feeling	dythymia	
thymo	thymus gland	thymocyte	
thymo		thymoma	
thyro	thyroid	thyroglobulin	
thyro		thyrotoxic (myopathy)	
toxi	poison	toxicant	
toxi		toxicology	
toxo	poison	toxoid	
tracheo	trachea	tracheocele	
tracheo		tracheolaryngotomy	
tracheo		tracheobronchitis	
thacheo		thacheorrhagia	
thacheo		thacheostenosis	
thacheo		thacheotomy	
trans	across, through	transdermal	
trans		transfusion	
trans		transplant	
trauma	accidental injury	traumatic delirium	
tri	three	tricuspid	
tri		trident	

Comprehensive Medical Thesaurus

Prefixes	Meanings	Examples	Meaning of Examples
trich	hair	trichitis	
trich		trichology	
trich		trichomycosis	
troph	food, nourishment	trophic	
tropho		trophoblastic cell	
tropho		trophology	
tropho		trophoneurosis	
tropho		trophonosis	
tropho		trophopathy	
typhlo	cecum	typhlostenosis	
typhlo		typhlotomy	
typhlo	blindness	typhlosis	
tyro	cheese	tyrogenous	
tyro		tyroma	
tyro		tyromatosis	
tyro		tyrosine	
tyro		tyrosis	

Section U

Prefixes	Meanings	Examples	Meaning of Examples
ultra	beyond	ultrasonic	
ultra		ultraviolet	
uric	uric acid	uricemia	
uric		uricosuria	
urin	urine	urinalysis	
urin		urinary	

Section V

Prefixes	Meanings	Examples	Meaning of Examples
vagi	vagina	vaginitis	
vagi		vaginopathy	
vagi		vaginoperineal	
vagi		vaginoperineotomy	
vagi		vaginotomy	
vagi		vaginovesical	
varico	bulging veins	varicose ulcer	
varico		varicosis	
varico		varicotomy	
vas	blood vessel	vasoconstriction	
vas		vasodilation	
vas		vasomotor	
veni	vein	venipuncture	
veno	vein	venotomy	
ventro	belly or front	ventrotomy	
vertebro	vertebral column	vertebrobasilar	
vertebro		vertebrocostal	
vesico	bladder	vesicoureteral	
vesico		vesicouterine	
vesico		vesicovaginal	

Section X

Prefixes	Meanings	Examples	Meaning of Examples
xeno	hetero, strange	xenogenesis	
xeno		xenograft	
xeno		xenoparasite	
xeno		xenophobia	
xeno		xenophonia	
xero	dry, dryness	xerochelia	
xero		xeroderma	
xero		xeroma	
xero		xerophthalmia	
xero		xeroradiography	
xero		xerostomia	

Section Z

Prefixes	Meanings	Examples	Meaning of Examples
zona	portion, belt	zonaglomerulosa	
zona	border	zonareticularis	
zone	local	zone therapy	
zone		zonesthesia	
zonul	ligament	zonulitis	
zonula	ligament	zonula cillaris	
zygo	union	zygosity	
zygo		zygote	
zymo	enzyme, fermentation	zymology	
zymo		zymosis	
zymo		zymotic disease	

CHAPTER 6

Suffixes by Alphabetical Order with Examples

Section A

Suffixes	Meanings	Examples	Meaning of Examples
adenoma	tumor	fibroadenoma	
agnosia	unable to perceive	paragnosia	
agogue	excite secretion	hormonagogue	
algesia	sensitivity to pain	hyperalgesia	
algia	pain	pleuralgia	
angina	severe pain - typically	herpangina	
angioma	blood vessel tumor	hemangioma	
anopia	defective vision	cyanopia	
anopsia	defective vision	hemianopsia	
anthem	eruption, rash	enanthem	
anthem		exanthem	
aphrodisia	sexual arousal	anaphrodisia	
asthenia	loss of vitality	neurasthenia	
atonia	atony, weak tension	myatonia	
auxe	growth	prostatauxe	

Comprehensive Medical Thesaurus

Section B

Suffixes	Meanings	Examples	Meaning of Examples
biotic	life	para<u>biotic</u>	
blast	originating cell	leuco<u>blast</u>	
blast	embryonic state	megaro<u>blast</u>	

Section C

Suffixes	Meanings	Examples	Meaning of Examples
cardia	heart condition	brachy<u>cardia</u>	
cardia		myo<u>cardia</u>	
cele	swelling, tumor	hydro<u>cele</u>	
cenosis	expel	pyo<u>cenosis</u>	
centesis	perforation, puncture	amnio<u>centesis</u>	
chezia	defecation	hemato<u>chezia</u>	
chrome	color	cyto<u>chrome</u>	
chylia	digestive juice	hypo<u>chylia</u>	
cide	kill	sui<u>cide</u>	
clasia	crushing operation	osteo<u>clasia</u>	
cle	small	parti<u>cle</u>	
clonus	spasm	myo<u>clonus</u>	
colon	part of intestine	sigmoid<u>colon</u>	
coria	condition of pupil	aniso<u>coria</u>	
cyst	fluid filled	myelo<u>cyst</u>	

Suffixes	Meanings	Examples	Meaning of Examples
cyte	cell	erythrocyte	
cyte		leucocyte	
cyte		lipocytes	

Section D

Suffixes	Meanings	Examples	Meaning of Examples
dendron	treelike formation	neurodendron	
derm	skin	angioderm	
dermic	related to the skin	hypodermic	
desis	bind, tie together	arthrodesis	
dilator	opening of passage	vasodilator	
diplopia	double vision	amphodiplopia	
dorsal	back of something	ventrodorsal	
dynia	pain	neurodynia	

Section E

Suffixes	Meanings	Examples	Meaning of Examples
ectasia	dilation, extension	ureterectasia	
ectasis	dilation	atelectasis	
ectasis		bronchiectasis	
ectasis		gastrectasis	
ectomy	cut out	nephrectomy	
ectomy		prostatectomy	
edema	swelling	lymphedema	
edema		papilledema	
emesis	vomiting	hematemesis	
emia	blood condition	anemia	
emia		hypercholesterolemia	
emia		hyperemia	
emia		hyperglycemia	
emia		hyperlipidemia	
emia		hypoglycemia	
emia		metremia	
emia		septicemia	
emia		uricemia	
esis	action, process result	synthesis	
esthesia	feeling, sensation	anesthesia	

Section F

Suffixes	Meanings	Examples	Meaning of Examples
fibroma	tumor, fibrous tissue	neurofibroma	

Section G

Suffixes	Meanings	Examples	Meaning of Examples
gamous	type of marriage	monogamous	
gamy	type of marriage	monogamy	
gastric	part of stomach	endogastric	
gen	generate	androgen	
gen	generate antibody	antigen	
gen	origin, formation	carcinogen	
genic	forming, causing, producing	bronchogenic	
genesis	produce, origin	thermogenesis	
glia	binding, glue	neuroglia	
globin	oxygen rich blood	hemoglobin	
gnosis	knowledge	diagnosis	
gram	drawing	cardiogram	
gram		echocardiogram	
graph	drawing	micrograph	

Section H

Suffixes	Meanings	Examples	Meaning of Examples
hidrosis	sweat	anhidrosis	
hidrosis		hyperhidrosis	
hypnia	sleep, hypnosis	anhypnia	

Section I

Suffixes	Meanings	Examples	Meaning of Examples
ia	specified condition	dysopia	
ia	poor health	hypoglycemia	
iasis	disease	lithiasis	
iasis		psoriasis	
ic	agent, drug	hypoglycemic	
ism	condition, theory	hypothyroidism	
ism		hyperthyroidism	
ist	one who does it	endocrinologist	
ist		gynecologist	
ite	body	hermaphrodite	
ite	compound	nitrite	
itis	inflammation	arthritis	
itis		bronchitis	
itis		bursitis	
itis		carditis	

Suffixes	Meanings	Examples	Meaning of Examples
itis	inflammation	cellulitis	
itis		cholangitis	
itis		cholecystitis	
itis		endocarditis	
itis		gastritis	
itis		hepatitis	
itis		meningitis	
itis		myelitis	
itis		pharyngitis	
itis		proctitis	
itis		proctocolitis	
itis		retinitis	
itis		rhinitis	
itis		sialadenitis	
itis		sinusitis	
itis		tendinitis	
ize	treatment	catheterize	

Section L

Suffixes	Meanings	Examples	Meaning of Examples
lalia	speech	echolalia	
lepsy	seizure	narcolepsy	
lith	calculus	gastrolith	
lith		pneumolith	
logy	science, study	cytology	
logy		physiology	
logy		proctology	
logy		serology	
lysis	break up, dissolution	blastolysis	
lysis	break down	cytolysis	
lysis		osteolysis	
lysis	blood cleaning	dialysis	
lyte	decomposed result	electrolyte	
lytic	decomposition	leucolytic	

Section M

Suffixes	Meanings	Examples	Meaning of Examples
malacia	softening	osteomalacia	
mania	mental disorder	enosimania	
maniac	crazy interest	narcomaniac	
maniac		kleptomaniac	
megaly	enlargement	cardiomegaly	
mentia	mind condition	dementia	
metry	measurement	acoumetry	
mia	disorder	achromia	
mia		agenosomia	
mia		dysthymia	
morph	form, structure	metamorphosis	
mucous	viscous secretions	seromucous	
mycin	antibiotics	streptomycin	
mycosis	fungus disease	blastomycosis	

Section N

Suffixes	Meanings	Examples	Meaning of Examples
nephric	related to kidney	peri<u>nephric</u>	
nesia	poor growth	age<u>nesia</u>	
neural	related to nerve	epi<u>neural</u>	
neural		myo<u>neural</u>	
neurotic	abnormal nerve	angio<u>neurotic</u>	
neurotic		vaso<u>neurotic</u>	

Section O

Suffixes	Meanings	Examples	Meaning of Examples
oid	form	blast<u>oid</u>	
oid	resembling something	myx<u>oid</u>	
oid	shape	spher<u>oid</u>	
oma	tumor	adi<u>poma</u>	
oma		angi<u>oma</u>	
oma		carcin<u>oma</u>	
oma		encephal<u>oma</u>	
oma		heapt<u>oma</u>	
oma		lymphangi<u>oma</u>	
oma		neuroangi<u>oma</u>	
oma		papill<u>oma</u>	
opia	defective vision	asthen<u>opia</u>	

Suffixes	Meanings	Examples	Meaning of Examples
opia	defective vision	hyper<u>opia</u>	
opia		my<u>opia</u>	
opia		nictal<u>opia</u>	
opia		protan<u>opia</u>	
ophthalmia	defective vision	ex<u>ophthalmia</u>	
opsia	visul condition	my<u>opsia</u>	
osis	condition	athiamin<u>osis</u>	
osis	action, process	diagn<u>osis</u>	
osis	pathological condition	endometri<u>osis</u>	
osis		hemochromat<u>osis</u>	
osis		narc<u>osis</u>	
osmia	sense of smell	dys<u>osmia</u>	
osmia		mer<u>osmia</u>	
oxia	cellular oxygen	an<u>oxia</u>	
oxia	condition of oxygen	hyp<u>oxia</u>	

COMPREHENSIVE MEDICAL THESAURUS

SECTION P

Suffixes	Meanings	Examples	Meaning of Examples
path	patient	psychopath	
pathy	illness, suffering	cardiomyopathy	
pathy		nephropathy	
pathy		osteopathy	
pathy		psychopathy	
pathy		splenopathy	
ped	foot	biped	
penia	deficiency	glycopenia	
penia		leukopenia	
penia		lipopenia	
penia		thrombocytopenia	
penia		thyropenia	
pepsia	state of digestion	anapepsia	
pepsia		dyspepsia	
pepsia		oligopepsia	
peptic		dyspeptic	
pexis	fixation	glycopexis	
pexis		hemopexis	
pexy	fixation	cardiomyopexy	
pexy		splenopexy	

Suffixes	Meanings	Examples	Meaning of Examples
phage	eating	hemophage	
phage		macrophage	
phagia	swallow	dysphagia	
phagia		bradyphagia	
phagy	eating	bacteriophagy	
phasia	speech disorder	aphasia	
phasia		dysphasia	
phemia		dysphemia	
philia	abnormal craving	necrophilia	
philia	excess amount	neutrophilia	
philia	tendency to act	spasmophilia	
phobe	fear	heliophobe	
phobia	abnormal fear	aerophobia	
phobia		agoraphobia	
phobia		necrophobia	
phobic	exhibiting fear	zoophobic	
phoria	condition	dysphoria	
phoria		euphoria	
phony	sound	echophony	
phrenia	mental disorder	schizophrenia	
phyma	swelling, tumor	rhinophyma	
plakia	patches on mucus membrane	melanoplakia	

Suffixes	Meanings	Examples	Meaning of Examples
plakia	patches	leukoplakia	
plasia	formation, development	hyperplasia	
plasm	cell or tissue	cytoplasm	
plasma	cell or tissue	mycoplasma	
plast	forming cell	lipoplast	
plast	originating cell	osteoplast	
plasty	reform, repair	angioplasty	
plasty	cosmetic	rhytidoplasty	
plasty	shaping	rhinoplasty	
plegia	paralysis	hemiplegia	
plegia		paraplegia	
plex	network, bundle	veniplex	
plexia	damage	pagoplexia	
plexy	stroke	apoplexy	
pnea	breath	branchypnea	
poietic	development, formation	hemopoietic	
pragia	quality of action	miopragia	
praxia	activity	hypopraxia	
ptosis	falling	esophagoptosis	
ptosis		cecoptosis	
ptysis	spitting	hemoptysis	

Section R

Suffixes	Meanings	Examples	Meaning of Examples
rhythmia	heart beat	brady<u>rhythmia</u>	
rhythmia		dys<u>rhythmia</u>	
rrhage	fluid, discharge	hemo<u>rrhage</u>	
rrhagia	discharge	meno<u>rrhagia</u>	
rrhea	fluid discharge	dia<u>rrhea</u>	
rrhexis	rupture	cardio<u>rrhexis</u>	
rrhinia	condition of nose	a<u>rrhinia</u>	
rrhoid	vein rupture	hemo<u>rrhoid</u>	

Section S

Suffixes	Meanings	Examples	Meaning of Examples
sarcoma	malignant neoplasm	angio<u>sarcoma</u>	
scapula	shoulder blade	meso<u>scapula</u>	
sclerosis	hardening	osteo<u>sclerosis</u>	
scope	observing instruments	angio<u>scope</u>	
scope		arthro<u>scope</u>	
scope		broncho<u>scope</u>	
scope		endo<u>scope</u>	
scope		fiber<u>scope</u>	
scope		hystero<u>scope</u>	
scope		laparo<u>scope</u>	

Comprehensive Medical Thesaurus

Suffixes	Meanings	Examples	Meaning of Examples
scope	observing instruments	laryngoscope	
scope		mediastinoscope	
scope		proctoscope	
scope		sigmoidoscope	
sia	specified condition	presbyopsia	
sialia	saliva	asialia	
sis	disorders	actinomycosis	
sis		bronchiectasis	
sis		cholechromyerosis	
sis		cholelithiasis	
sis		endometriosis	
sis		fibrosis	
sis		hydronephrosis	
sis		hypochondriasis	
sis		lymphomatosis	
sis		microlithiasis	
sis		neurosis	
sis		osmidrosis	
sis		osteoporosis	
sis		otomycosis	
sis		pancreatolithiasis	
sis		pneumoconiosis	

Suffixes	Meanings	Examples	Meaning of Examples
sis	disorders	poliosis	
sis		proctostasis	
sis		prosthesis	
sis		psoriasis	
sis		psychosis	
sis		sclerosis	
sis		sepsis	
sis		spondylosis	
sis		stenosis	
sis		thrombosis	
sitia	appetite	eusitia	
some	body	chromosome	
somia	condition of the body	agenosomia	
somnia	sleep	insomnia	
spasm	convulsion	gastrospasm	
spasm		neurospasm	
spasm		vasospasm	
spermia	producing	aspermia	
stasia	ability to stand	dysstasia	
stasis	stoppage	hemostasis	
stasis		menostasis	
steoma	bone tumor	endosteoma	

COMPREHENSIVE MEDICAL THESAURUS

Suffixes	Meanings	Examples	Meaning of Examples
stomy	surgical opening	colostomy	
stomy		gastrostomy	
stomy	surgical opening	ileostomy	
stomy		ureterostomy	
stomy		urostomy	

SECTION T

Suffixes	Meanings	Examples	Meaning of Examples
thelia	condition of nipples	polythelia	
thelia		microthelia	
therapy	medical treatment	chemotherapy	
therapy		gonadotherapy	
therapy		immunotherapy	
therapy		pharmacotherapy	
thoracic	chest	intrathoracic	
thymia	feeling	dysthymia	
tome	cutting instrument	dermatome	
tome		neurotome	
tomy	incision	cystotomy	
tomy		hysteromyotomy	
tomy		laparotomy	
tomy		myotomy	

256

Suffixes	Meanings	Examples	Meaning of Examples
tomy	incision	myringotomy	
tomy		phlebotomy	
tomy		rhizotomy	
tonia	stress disorder	myotonia	
tonia	tonus	myatonia	
tonic	drug, muscle quality	cardiactonic	
tonic	solution concentration	hypotonic	
toxemia	infected poison	endotoxemia	
toxemia		gonotoxemia	
tresia	perforation	atresia	
tribe	crushing tool	angiotribe	
trichia	hair condition	leukotrichia	
trophic	type of nutrition	lipotrophic	
trophy	nourishment	atrophy	
trophy		dystrophy	
tropic	influence	radiotropic	
tropy	affinity, influence	syntropy	

Section U

Suffixes	Meanings	Examples	Meaning of Examples
ular	resembling	circular	
ular		tubular	
ulent	full of	feculent	
ulent		pulverulent	
ulent		succulent	
uria	urine	hematuria	
uria		nocturia	
uria		proteinuria	

Section V

Suffixes	Meanings	Examples	Meaning of Examples
vaccine	immunity to diseases	heterovaccine	
vert	turning	avert	
vert	turning direction	introvert	
vert		invert	

CHAPTER 7

LINGUISTIC ANALYSIS OF MEDICAL THESAURUS

In this chapter, some examples of identical meanings with different prefixes and suffixes are edited. Thesaurus is a group of words simply related to each other, but not necessarily identical.

Example 1: Erythrocythemia

    Erythro<u>cythemia</u> (increased red blood cells)

    Erythro<u>cytosis</u> (the same as above)

    Poly<u>cythemia</u> (the same as above)

Table 1: Linguistic Analysis of Example 1

Prefixes	Meanings	Suffixes	Meaning
cyt	cell	cyte	cell
cyto	cell	cythemia	condition of blood cell
erythrocyte	red blood cell	emia	condition of blood
erythro	red	ia	disorder
poly	many	osis	disorder

Example 2: Ablepsy and Myopia

<u>A</u><u>blepsy</u> or <u>A</u><u>blepsia</u> (blind)   My<u>opia</u> (nearsighted)

<u>An</u><u>opia</u> or <u>An</u><u>opsia</u> (blind)   My<u>opy</u> (nearsighted)

<u>Typhlo</u>sis (blind)   My<u>opsia</u> (nearsighted)

<u>A</u>chromat<u>opsia</u> (colorblind)   My<u>opsy</u> (nearsighted)

Table 2: Linguistic Analysis of Example 2

Prefixes	Meanings	Suffixes	Meaning
a	negative	blepsia	sight
an	negative	blepsy	sight
typhlo	blindness	opia	visual condition
my	muscle	opsia	visual condition
		opsy	visual condition
		opy	visual condition

Example 3: Poor Blood Supply (General or Heart)

<u>General</u>

Anemia (lack of blood supply)

Hypoemia (same)

Ischemia (same)

Pancytopenia (lack of cellular elements)

<u>Heart Blood Vessel Stenosis</u>

Angina pectoris

Stenocardia

Table 3: Linguistic Analysis of Example 3

Prefixes	Meanings	Stems	Meanings	Suffixes	Meanings
an	deficiency	isch	poor blood	cardia	heart
angi	blood vessel	pancyto	cellular elements of the blood	emia	blood condition
hypo	deficiency			hemia	blood condition
steno	narrow			penia	deficiency

Example 4: Insomnia (lack of sleep) most commonly in use

    Agrypnea*   (   ) *Obsolete terminology

    Anhypnea   (   )

    Anhypnosis   (   )

    Insomnia   (   ) hyposomnia

Table 4: Analysis of Example 4

Prefixes	Meanings	Suffixes	Meaning
an	not	ia	state of
in	not	sis	disorder
a	not	pnea	breath
hypo	lack of	somnus (somnia)	sleep

Example 5: Malnutrition (   )

    Atrophy (poor nutrition)

    Dystrophy (same)

    Malnutrition (same)

Table 5: Linguistic Analysis of Example 5

Prefixes	Meanings	Suffixes	Meaning
a	negative	trophy	nourishment
dys	negative	nutrition	nourishment
mal	poor		

Example 6: Atelo, Keno   imperfect, incomplete

    Atelocardia (imperfect heart development)

    Kenogenesis (incomplete development)

Table 6: Linguistic Analysis of Example 6

Prefixes	Meanings	Suffixes	Meaning
atelo	incomplete	cardia	heart
keno	empty	genesis	development

Example 7: Achalasia, Myotonia

    Achalasia (no relaxation)

    Atony (loss of tension)

    Myotonia (contraction of muscle)

    Dystonia (contraction of muscle)

    Table 7: Linguistic Analysis of Example 7

Prefixes	Meanings	Suffixes	Meaning
a	not or no	chalasia	relaxation
dys	bad	tony	tension, condition
mao	muscle	tonia	contraction

Example 8: Achylous and Achlorhydria

    Table 8: Analysis of Stems

    Chylous (gastric juice)

    Chlorhydria (gastric juice)

Example 9: Aethenia, Asthenia, Adynamic

    Aethenia (poor strength, weakness)

    Asthenia (poor strength)

    Adynamic (poor strength)

    Myasthenia (muscle weakness)

Table 9: Analysis

ethenia (strength)

dynamic (strength)

my (muscle)

sthenia (strength)

Example 10: Reproduction

<u>Gametogenesis</u>

<u>Gamogenesis</u>

<u>Oogamy</u>

<u>Oogenesis</u>

Ovario<u>cyesis</u>

Salpingo<u>cyesis</u>

Spermato<u>genesis</u>

Table 10: Linguistic Analysis of Example 10

Prefixes	Meanings	Suffixes	Meaning
gamo	marriage	cyesis	pregnancy
gameto	reproduction cell	gamy	fertilization
oo	oocyte	genesis	production

Example 11: Bleeding, Excretion

    Hemorrhage   Diarrhea

    Hemoptysis   Hidrorrhea

    Hemorrhoid   Hysterorrhea

    Menorrhea   Sialorrhea

    Menorrhagia

Table 11: Linguistic Analysis of Example 11

Prefixes	Meanings	Suffixes	Meaning
dia	apart, through	ptysis	spitting
hemo	blood	rrhage	flow, discharge
hystero	uterus	rrhagia	discharge
meno	blood and tissue	rrhea	flow discharge
sialo	saliva	rrhoid	varicosity (vein bleeding)

Example 12: Arrhythmia, Dysrhythmia

    a) Identical meaning related to heart rhythm

        Anisosphygmia

        Arrhythmia

        Dysrhythmia

Table 12a: Analysis of above examples

a (negative meaning)

aniso (dissimilar, unequal)

dys (negative, difficult)

ia (suffix for disorder)

rhythm

sphygm (pulse)

b) Not identical thesaurus related to heart rhythm disorder

Contraction	brachy cardia
Fibrillation	brady cardia
Flutter	

Example 13: Thesaurus-related Muscular Atrophy*

a) Muscular Atrophy: This is a motor neuron dysfunction.

b) Muscular Dystrophy: This is a degeneration of neural tissue in the brain, which causes progressive insidious muscle dysfunction.

Thesaurus also related to Muscular Atrophy

    c) Amyotonia

    d) Amyotrophia

Comparison: Myotonia (stressed muscle)
                      Amyotonia (relaxed muscle)

---

*Note that "Muscular Atrophy" is a Latin and Greek combined terminology; also, "Muscular Dystrophy" is a combined Latin and Greek example. These are related but nonidentical thesaurus.

Amyotonia means weak muscle due to poor nourishment. This disorder is caused by motor dysfunction.

Amyotrophia is a degeneration of motor neuron due to poor nourishment called muscular atrophy. Amyotrophia is also called Amyotrophic Lateral Sclerosis (ALS).

Table 13: Linguistic Analysis of Example 13

Prefixes/Suffixes	Origin	Meaning
atonia	Greek	relaxed condition
atrophy	Greek	poor nourishment
musculus	Latin	muscular
myo	Greek	muscular
tonia	Greek	relaxed condition
tonos	Greek	tone
trophe	Greek	nourishment

Example 14: Oophoron and Ovary

   a) Identical Meaning

      Ovaritis and Oophoritis

      Ovariancyst and Oophorocystosis

Table 14a: Identical Thesaurus Example

Stems	Meaning	Suffixes	Meanings of Suffixes
ovary (ovum in Latin)	egg	itis	inflammation
oophoron (Greek)	egg	cystosis	cyst formation

b) Thesaurus with different suffixes. (Not identical meaning)

Table 14b: Example

Thesaurus	Suffixes	Meaning	Meaning of Thesaurus
oophorectomy	ectomy	surgical removal	
oophorocystosis	cystosis	cyst formation	
oophorosalpingectomy	ectomy	surgical removal	
ovariectomy	ectomy	surgical removal	
ovariocentesis	centesis	perforation or puncture	
ovariocyesis	cyesis	pregnancy	
ovariostomy	stomy	surgical opening	
ovariotomy	tomy	surgical incision	
salpingitis	itis	inflammation	
salpingocyesis	cyesis	pregnancy	
salpingoma	oma	tumor	
salpingopexia	pexia	fixation	
salpingostomy	stomy	surgical opening	

Note: Salpinx means "tube" in Greek. "Salping" in this case means "ovarian tube."

Example 15: Words related to Benign Prostate Disorders

The prostate enlargement in senior men is associated with the hormone called dihydrotestosterone (DHT). The prostate growth squeezes the urethra (   ) and interferes with the normal flow of urine, which causes pain during urination.

Table 15: Thesaurus for Prostate Growth

Prostat<u>auxe</u>

Prostato<u>megaly</u>

Prostate <u>Hypertrophy</u>

Prostat<u>ism</u>

Benign Prostatic <u>Hyperplasia</u> (BPH)

Benign Prostatic <u>Hypertrophy</u> (BPH)

Note: Some of the above are no longer commonly used.

<u>Table 15: Linguistic Analysis of Example 15</u>

auxe	growth (auxein in Greek)
auxesis (Greek)	auxetic growth means hypertrophy
benign	means "noncancerous"
hyper	prefix for super or excess
mega	large in Greek
megaly	suffix for enlargement
plasia	suffix for formation or development
trophy	suffix for growth or nutrition

List of Thesaurus:

Prostatectomy

Prostatitis   This inflammation is caused by bacterial infection.

Prostatocystitis

Prostatovesiculitis

CHAPTER 8

Elemental Change of Location in Compound Words

Compound terminology consists of two or three elements and order of these elements can be located without any change of medical meaning. In other words, these words are called Identical Compound Thesaurus. Other examples are called Related Compound Thesaurus.

Example 1: Angio and Fibro
Identical Compound Thesaurus

<u>Angiofibro</u>ma

<u>Fibroangioma</u>

Related Compound Thesaurus

He<u>mangio</u>ma

<u>Hema</u>toma

Analysis of Example 1

    Angio --------- Aggeion (Greek)   blood vessel

    Fibro ---------- Fibra (Latin)   fiber

    Hem ---------- Haima (Greek)   blood

    Hemat ------- Haima   blood

    ma ------------ Oma (Greek)   tumor

Example 2: Fibro and Neuro

    Identical Compound Thesaurus

        Fibroneuroma

        Neurofibroma

    Related Compound Thesaurus

        Fibromyoma

Analysis of Example 2

Myo ---------- Myelos, Mys (Greek)		muscle
Neuro -------- Neuron (Greek)		nerve

Example 3: Cardio and Myo

    Cardiomyopathy

    Myocardial Infarction

    Myocarditis

Analysis of Example 3

Cardio ---------------- Kardia (Greek)	heart
Infarction ------------ Infarcire (Latin)	local tissue necrosis
Myo ------------------- Myelos (Greek)	muscle
Pathy ----------------- Pati (Latin)	suffer
Suffix ----------------- itis (Greek)	inflammation

Example 4: Cysto, Fibro and Neuro

    Fibro<u>cyto</u>ma

    <u>Neurocyto</u>ma

    <u>Neuro</u>ma

<u>Analysis of Example 4</u>

Cyto ------------------- Kytos (Greek)		cell
Cytoma ---------------- Oma (Greek)		tumor

Example 5: Fibro, Leio and Myo

    <u>Leiomyofibro</u>ma

    <u>Leiomyo</u>ma

    <u>Leiomyo</u>ma Uteri

<u>Analysis of Example 5</u>

Fibro ---------- Fibra (Latin)	fiber
Fibroma ------ Fibroid uteri	tumor in uterus
Leio ---------- Leios (Greek)	smooth
Myoma ------ Fibroid uteri	tumor in uterus

Example 6: Chondro, Osteo and Sarco

    Chondrosarcoma

    Fibrosarcoma

    Osteochondrosarcoma

    Osteogenic sarcoma

    Osteosarcoma

Analysis of Example 6

    Chondro ----- (Greek) ----- cartilage

    Fibro ---------- Fibra (Latin) ----- fiber

    Osteo --------- Osteon (Greek) ----- bone

    Sarco --------- Sarx (Greek) ----- flesh

Example 7: Lipo, Fibro and Sarco
    Identical Compound Thesaurus

        Fibrolipoma

        Lipofibroma

        Lipoma fibrosum

    Related Compound Thesaurus

        Fibrosarcoma

        Liposarcoma

Analysis of Example 7

    Lipo ----- Lipos (Greek) ----- fat

    Lipoma ----- oma (Greek) ----- fat tumor

Example 8: Cranial, Cerebro, Spinal, Spino

    Identical Compound Thesaurus

    Cerebrospinal nerves

    Spinocranial nerves

Spelling changes of Compound Thesaurus
    "al" changes to "o"

CHAPTER 9

Examples of Analogy Between Prefix and Suffix

Section A

Prefix	Suffix	Meaning	Example
angio		blood vessel	angioplasty
	angioma	vessel tumor	hem angioma
asthenic		no strength	asthenic habitus
	asthenia	no vitality	neurasthenia
auxe		growth	auxesis
	auxe	growth	prostatauxe
auxo		growth	auxocardia
auxo		growth	auxocyte

Section B

Prefix	Suffix	Meaning	Example
bio		life	bioscopy
	biotic	life	parabiotic
blast		embryonic	blastoma
	blast	originating	leucoblast

Section C

Prefix	Suffix	Meaning	Example	
cardia		heart disorder	cardiac arrest	
	cardia	heart disorder	myocardia	
cele		cavity	celectome	
	cele	cavity	celiocele	
	cele	cavity	tracheocele	
cell		cell	cellular	
cell		cell	cellulitis	
	cyte	cell	leucocyte	
cyto		cell	cytoplasm	
cephal		headache	cephalalgia	
	cephalia	headache	hemicephalia	
cerebral		brain	cerebralgia	
	cerebral	brain	postcerebral	
chroma		color	chromatopsia	
	chromia	color	orthochromia	
chroma		color	chromatosome	
	chromasia	color	hyperchromasia	
chromo		color	chromocyte	
	chromatic	color	panchromatic	
chromo		color	chromogen	

Prefix	Suffix	Meaning	Example	
colon		colon	colonalgia	
	colonic	colon	rectocolonic	
coma	coma	deep sleep	comatose	
		deep sleep	semicoma	

Section D

Prefix	Suffix	Meaning	Example	
dactylo		finger, toe	dactylospasm	
	dactylia	finger	ankylodactylia	
	derm	skin	angioderm	
derma		skin	dermatitis	
dermo		skin	dermotherapy	
dorso		back	dorsocephalad	
	dorsal	back	thoracodorsal	
	drome	runs in special disorder	syndrome	
dromo		runs in special disorder	dromomania	
dromo		runs in special disorder	dromotrope	

Section F

Prefix	Suffix	Meaning	Example	
fibro		fiber	fibroadenoma	
	fibroma	fibrous tumor	neurofibroma	

Section G

Prefix	Suffix	Meaning	Example	
gam		marriage	gamete	
	gamy	marriage	monogamy	
gastr		stomach	gastritis	
	gastr	stomach	endogastric	
gen		produce	generate	
	gen	produce	antigen	
gen		sex	genital	
	gen	sex	androgen	
genetic		origin	genetic	
	genetic	origin	gamogenetic	
	genital	sex	male genitals	
genito		sex	genitourinary	
glia		glue	glia cell	
	glia	glue	neuroglia	
	globin	small sphere	hemoglobin	
globul		small sphere	globulolysis	

Prefix	Suffix	Meaning	Example	
glyce		sweet	glycerin	
glyce		sweet	glycerol	
	glyce	sweet	hyperglycemia	

Section H

Prefix	Suffix	Meaning	Example	
hidro		sweat	hidrodermia	
hidro		sweat	hidrorrhea	
	hidrosis	sweat	anhidrosis	
hypno		sleep	hypnopathy	
	hypnia	sleep	anhypnia	
hypno		hypnosis	hypnotic	

Section L

Prefix	Suffix	Meaning	Example	
lalio		speech	laliophobia	
	lalia	speech	echolalia	
lith		stone	lithotomy	
	lith	stone	gastrolith	

Section M

Prefix	Suffix	Meaning	Example
muco		mucous	mucocele
	mucous	mucous	fibromucous

Section P

Prefix	Suffix	Meaning	Example
peps		digestion	pepsin
	pepsia	digestion	anapepsia
phago	phage	eating	macrophage
	phagia	swallow	dysphagia
		eating	phagocyte
plasma	plasm	blood cell	cytoplasm
		blood cell	plasmacytoma
	plasma	blood cell	mycoplasma
plex		strike	plexor
	plex	network (nerve)	neuroplexus
	plex	network (vein)	veniplex
poie		development	poiesis
	poie	development	hemopoietic
pneumo	pnea	breathing	brachypnea
		breathing	pneumodynamics

Prefix	Suffix	Meaning	Example	
pneumo		lung	pneumocele	
	pneumonia	lung disorder	pleuropneumonia	
potent		ability	potentiate	
	potent	ability	unipotent	
	prosopia	face	ateloprosopia	
prosopo		face	prosopoplegia	
psych		mind	psychosis	
	phychic	mind	allopsychic	
puer		child	puerperal	
puer		child	puerperal fever	
pueri		child	puericulture	
	puerility	childish	puerility	

Section S

Prefix	Suffix	Meaning	Example	
seps		decay	sepsometer	
	sepsis	decay	typhosepsis	
	sepsis	decay	urosepsis	
	septic	decay	antiseptic	
septice		decay	septicemia	
sialo		saliva	sialogogue	
sialo		saliva	sialorrhea	
	sialia	saliva	asialia	
	sitia	appetite	eusitia	
sito		food	sitology	
somni		sleep	somnipathy	
	somnia	sleep	hyposomnia	
spasm		convulsion	spasmodermia	
	spasm	convulsion	bronchospasm	
	sphere	sphere	somosphere	
sphero		sphere	spherocyte	
sphygm		pulse	sphygmometer	
	sphygmia	pulse	anisosphygmia	
splen		spleen	splenectomy	
	splenia	spleen	asplenia	

Prefix	Suffix	Meaning	Example
spore		seed	sporicide
	spore	seed	archespore
	sternia	sternum bone	schistosternia
sterno		sternum bone	sternocostal
stoma		mouth	stomatopathy
stoma		mouth	stomatitis
	stomia	mouth	atelostomia

Section T

Prefix	Suffix	Meaning	Example
	thyrea	thyroid	hypothyrea
thyro		thyroid	thyroid hormone
tomo	tome	cutting	pleurotome
		cutting	tomography
	tomy	cutting	oncotomy
toxe		poison	toxemia
	toxia	poison	thyrotoxia
	toxic	poison	hemotoxic
toxo		poison	toxonosis
toxo		poison	toxoplasma

Section V

Prefix	Suffix	Meaning	Example	
	veni	vein	endo<u>ven</u>itis	
veno		vein	<u>ven</u>otomy	
ventral		belly	<u>ventral</u> hernia	
	ventral		dorso<u>ventral</u>	
ventri		small cavity	<u>ventri</u>cle	
vert		back	<u>vert</u>ebra	
	verse	turn	re<u>verse</u>	

Section Z

Prefix	Suffix	Meaning	Example	
zymo		fermentation	<u>zymo</u>logy	
	zyme	enzyme	en<u>zyme</u>	
	zyme		lyso<u>zyme</u>	

PART III

QUICK OVERVIEW OF ASSOCIATED MEDICAL THESAURUS

Chapter 1. Thesaurus Relating Psychoneurotic Disorders

Mental Disorder
Psychosis

Neurotic Disorder
Neurosis

Psychoneurotic
Hypochondriasis
Psychosomatic

Agnosia or Agnosis
Autotopagnosia
Auto-image Agnosis

Anorexia Nervosa
Anxiety Neurosis
Anxiety Psychosis

Compulsive Neurosis
Obsessive Neurosis

Anhypnia
Insomnia

Delusion
Hallucination

Palsy
Paralysis

Paranoia
Schizophrenia
Catatonia
Catatonic Schizophrenia
Latent Schizophrenia
Paranoid Schizophrenia
Reactive Schizophrenia
Residual Schyzophrenia

Mental Deficiency
Mental Retardation
Down's Syndrome

Chapter 2. Blood Pressure-related Thesaurus and Glossary

ACE inhibitors (Angiotensin-Converting Enzyme Inhibitors):
   Drugs to prevent the formation of "angiotensin."

Angiotensin:
   A polypeptide (chain of amino acids) in the blood causing vasoconstriction.

Antiadrenergics:
   Drugs to reduce the muscle tone in peripheral blood vessels.

Anticoagulants:
   To prevent clot formation. To prevent vein thrombosis.

Atrial fibrillation:
   Heart rhythm abnormality

Beta-Blockers (Beta Adrenergic Blockers):
   Reduce the heart rate and also relieve the pain of angina.

Calcium Channel-Blockers:
   Drugs used for vasodilation, relaxing muscle cells of the blood vessels.

Digitalis Glycosides:
   To control irregular heart rhythm.

Diuretics (or Water Pills):
   Drugs used to remove water from the bloodstream and to reduce blood pressure.

Nitrates:
   Drugs for the relief of angina pectoris pain, to keep up with the heart's demand for oxygen.

Thrombolytics (Clot Busters):
   Drugs to dissolve clots in the blood vessels, and also in the lungs causing pulmonary emboli.

Vasodilators:
   Drugs used to lower blood pressure when other drugs have not been effective, depending on disorders.

Surgical Treatments:
    Artery Bypass Surgery (or Grafting)
        A shunt to bypass a blocked artery.
    Heart Valve Replacement

Chapter 3. Respiratory-related Therapeutic Thesaurus

Adrenergics:
    Drugs improve air flow into the lungs and relieve nasal congestion.

Bronchodilators:
    Relax the smooth muscles of the respiratory passages.

Corticosteroids:
    Hormones produced by the body, associated with the adrenal cortex. They, are either natural or drugs, and fight inflammatin and also regulate the immune system.
Cough Suppressants
Spirometry Treatment

<u>Types of Lung Surgery</u>

    a.) Tracheotomy:
        A tube is inserted through the opening to remove secretions and allow the passage of air.
    b.) Lobectomy
    c.) Pneumoectomy
    d.) Segmental Resection
    e.) Wedge Resection

Chapter 4. Dietary-related Thesaurus

Dietetics:
    Study of diet and nutrition.

Dietitian:
    Registered diet expert.
    Diet Technician
    People who have an associate degree.
    Calorie-related diet

Dietary Allowance:
    An official guide for essential nutrients.

Dietary Fiber

Metabolic-related Thesaurus

Antacids:
    To reduce acidity in the digestive tract.

Antilipidemic:
    To reduce levels of fat content.
    Low-Cholesterol Diet
    Low-Fat Diet

Fiber-Modified Diet:
    It helps eliminate body wastes.

Gluten-Free Diet:
    It helps prevent diarrhea, vomiting, malnutrition, weight loss.

Low-Purine Diet:
    Prevention of gout and kidney stones formation.

Low-Salt Diet:
    It helps correct water retention and swelling.

Lactose-Reduced Diet:
    Treatment of lactose intolerance caused by dairy products.

High-Protein Diet:
    It helps individual gain weight and feel stronger and also resist infections.
    Mineral Supplements

Hyperkalemia:
    Excess potassium in the blood due to renal failure.

Chapter 5. Vitamin-related Thesaurus

Carotenoid (or called beta-carotene)
   This is a potent source of Vitamin.

Niacin (or called Nicotinic Acid)
   Manufacture of healthy skin and sex hormone.

Pantothenic Acid
   Produce corticosteroids, sex hormones and healthy skin.

Vitamin A (or called Beta Carotene)
   Essential for strong bones, teeth, and healthy skin.
   Help treat eye problems and skin disorders.

Vitamin B (or Thiamin)
   This is water soluble and essential for metabolism

Vitamin B6 (Pyridoxin)
   Produce red blood cells and antibodies.

Vitamin B12 (or Cyanocobalamin)
   Help reduce depression. This is important in the production of
   genetic substances.

Vitamin Complex (or B-Complex as a trade mark)
   Metabolism of carbohydrates, fats and protein.
   Vital role in the activities of various enzymes.

Vitamin C (Ascorbic Acid)
   Important for growth of healthy bones, teeth, ligaments, blood vessels.

Vitamin D: Soluble in fat called Steatolysis (see Chapter 16)
   Similar to Vitamin C
      D2 (Ergocalciferol)
      D3 (Cholecalciferol)

Vitamin E
   Important for normal cell structure. Extra vitamin E produce more antibodies and bolster seniors' ability to fight infection. It may slow aging problems. (see page 310)

Vitamin K
   It helps prevent blood clotting, hemorrhaging, build strong bones.

Chapter 6. Glossary Related to Natural Medicine

Acupressure:
   A method of anesthesia, also called shiatsu.

Acupuncture:
   Another method of analgesia by inserting needles.

Ayurveda:
   This is a change of lifestyle originated in India.

Exercise Therapy
   Relaxation

Homeopathy (Holistic health care)
   Aromatherapy
   Essence therapy
   Herb therapy
   Juice therapy
   Mineral therapy

Massage:
   Rubbing and kneading to relieve painful muscle spasm.

Yoga:
   It releases built-up tension and stress.

Zen-shiatsu:
   This is a strenuous practice with heavy pressue and Yoga-like stretches, originated in Japan.

Miscellaneous therapy
   Hydrotherapy
   Imagery
   Meditation

Chapter 7. Examples of Pseudothesaurus

"Pseud" means "false," originating from Greek "Pseudes."

A) *Group of Thesaurus with Pseudo or Pseud*
Pseudoanemia

Pseudoangina

Pseudarthrosis

Pseudesthesia

Pseudoataxia

Pseudocataract

Pseudochylous Ascites

Pseudocyesis

Pseudocyst

Pseudodementia

Pseudoephedrine (Decongestant drug to relieve nasal congestion)

Pseudoepidemic (Sick building syndrome)

Pseudohermaphoroditism (External genitalia resemble opposite sex)

Pseudomeningitis

Pseudoneumonia

Pseudopregnancy

Pseudotumor

B) *Group of Associated Thesaurus (Acute, Benign, Latent, Pseudo)*

Acute dementia (Impaired cognitive function)

Pseudodementia

Latent Schizophrenia

Pseudoneurotic Schizophrenia

Pseudopsychopathic Schizophrenia

Membrane (Membrana means thin skin in Latin.)

Pseudomembrane

Pseudomembranous

C) *Group of Identical Thesaurus*

Pseudocyesis

Pseudopregnancy

D) *Pseudotumor cerebri*

Benign intracranial hypertension

Benign brain tumor

Meningioma

Chapter 8. Thesaurus Relating Advanced Diagnostic Systems

"Signa Profile" MRI System
  Developed by G.E. Medical Systems ("—-" indicates Trade Name)

Neuroimaging "Signa" SP System
  Developed for intraoperative surgery by G.E.

"HighSpeed" CT System
  Subsecond imaging capability

"Advantx Legacy" DR & F System
  Versatile digital imaging

"LOGIQ" 700 MR System
  MD digital ultrasound platform

"Optima" NX Dual-head System
  Nuclear imaging system

See also Part I, Chapter 5: Thesaurus of Medical Technology

Chapter 9. Thesaurus Relating "Cata-" or "Meta-"

a) *Cata:* This prefix means "breakdown."

   Catabiosis

   Catabolism

   Catastrophe

   Catastrophic Reaction

   Catatonia

   Catatonic Excitement

   Catatonic Stupor

   Catatonic Schizophrenia

   Catalepsy

   Cataplexy

b) *Meta:* This prefix means "exchange" or "change."

   Metagenesis

   Metaphases

   Metaplasia

   Metaplasm

   Metastasis

   Mitosis

c) *Metabolism*

   Metabolic Disorder

   Metabolite

   Metabolic Acidosis

   Metabolic Alkalosis

Chapter 10. Thesaurus Relating Hormones

a) *Group of Pituitary Hormones*

    Adrenocorticotropic Hormone (ACTH)

    Somatropic Hormone (STH)

    Follicle-Stimulating Hormone (FSH)

    Lutenizing Hormone (LH)

    Progesterone

    Prolactine

    Progesterone

    Estrogen

    Antidiuretic Hormone or Vasopressin

    Oxytocin

b) *Group of Hormones Relating Thyroid (see also pgs. 300 and 301)*

    Thyroxine

    Thyrotropin-Releasing Hormone (TRH)

    Parathyroid Hormone (PTH)

    Calcitonin

c) *Group of Gonadal Hormones*

    Gonadotropin Hormone

    Ovarian Hormone

    Lutenizing Hormone (LH)

    Estrogen (or Progesterone)

    Testosterone

Androgen

d) *Group of Adrenal Hormones*

Steroid

Anabolic Steroid

Corticotropin (ACTH)

Aldosterone

e) *Group of Renal Hormones*

Erythropoietin (EPO)

Aldosterone Adrenal Hormone

f) *Group of Pancreatic and Gastrointestinal Hormones*

Insulin

Gastrin

Glucagon

Polypeptide Hormone

Chapter 11. Thesaurus Relating Enzymes (or Protein Metabolism)

a) *Various Types of Enzyme*

Amylase

Coenzyme: This is an additional component supplied by a vitamin.

Lipase

Protease

Protein Kinase

b) *Group by Manufacturing Origins*

Comprehensive Medical Thesaurus

Extracellular Enzyme

Intracellular Enzyme

Digestive Enzyme: Release more than others and catalyze chemical reactions.

Liver Enzyme

Muscle Enzyme

Pancreatic Enzyme

Heart Enzyme: Heart muscle cells release enzymes, particularly more after a myocardial infarction.

c) *Group of Enzymes by Biochemical Reaction, Catalyze Reaction*

Autolytic Enzyme

Coagulating Enzyme

Deaminating Enzyme

Glycolytic Enzyme

Hydrolytic Enzyme

Inverting Enzyme

Lipolytic Enzyme

Oxidative Enzyme

Proteolytic Enzyme

Reducing Enzyme

Steatolytic Enzyme

Uricolytic Enzyme

d) *Group of Disorders Relating Enzyme (See also (g))*

Enzymatic Detergent Asthma

Enzymosis

Enzymuria (also called Albuminuria or Proteinuria)

e) *Protein Synthesis*

DNA: Deoxyribonucleic Acid

DNA Ligase: an Enzyme to repair a strand of DNA.

DNA Polymerase: an Enzyme to catalyze DNA.

Genetic Code

Genetic Engineering

Genetic Equilibrium

Genetic Homeostasis

RNA: Ribonucleic Acid

RNA Polymerase

RNA Splicing

f) *Enzyme-linked Assay Test*

ELISA: Enzyme-linked Immunosorbent Assay
This is to test the presence or absence in the blood of a specific protein such as antigen or antibody.

g) *Genetic Disorders Caused by Abnormal Enzyme in the Blood*

G6PD Deficiency: Inherited abnormal red blood cells.

Galactosemia: Due to the absence of an enzyme in the liver.

12. Thesaurus Relating the Thyroid Gland

a) *Suffix relating condition of the gland*

-thyrea

-thyreosis

-thyroidism

b) *Hyperthyroidism*

Goiter

Grave's Disease

Hashimoto's Disease

c) *Hypothyroidism*

Myxedema: Swelling of the hands, face and feet.

d) *Cancer, tumor*

Thyroid cancer

Thyrophyma

e) *Miscellaneous*

Thyroiditis

Thyrotoxicosis

Thyrotoximyopathy

Thyrotoxin

f) *Surgical*

Thyroidectomy

Thyrotomy

Thyrochondrotomy

g) *Thyroid Hormone*

Thyroxine (T4)

Tridothyroxine (T3)

Thyroid-Stimulating Hormone (TSH)

Thyrotropin-Releasing Hormone (TRH)

Chapter 13. Thesaurus Relating Blood Disorders

a) *White Blood Cell Disorder*

Acute Myelocytic Leukemia
   Myelogenous cells—Mutation—Excess White Blood Cells
Acute Lymphocytic Leukemia
   Lymphogenous cells—Mutation—Excess White Blood Cells

Chronic Myelogenous Leukemia

Chronic Granulocytic Lukemia

Hodgkin's Lymphoma—Malignant Lymphoid

b) *Red Blood Cells*

Bone Marrow makes normal blood cells.

Sickle Cell Disease (Inherited disease)
   Sickle cells cause plugs in small blood vessels.

c) *Miscellaneous Blood Disorders*

Anemia

Aplastic Anemia

Hemolytic Anemia

Megaloblastic Anemia

Sickle Cell Anemia

Anemic Anoxia

Thrombocytopenia (A deficiency of platelets)

Cyanosis (Bluish discolor due to defect in the hemoglobin molecule)

Hypoglycemia (Glucopenia)

Hyperglycemia (Glycosemia)

Glycosuria (Glucosuria)

Hypermagnesemia

Hypomagnesemia

Hypocalcemia

Hypoxemia

Hypoxia

Granulocytosis

Iron-deficiency Anemia

Porphyria
    Atopic Porphyria
    Hepatic Porphyria

Purpura (Bleeding due to thrombocytopenia)

d) *AIDS (Acquired Immune Deficiency Syndrome)*

HIV: Human Immunodeficiency Virus

CD4: CD4 Positive Lymphocyte Count or T-4 Helper Count

e) *Hematopoietic Disorders due to AIDS*

Bone Marrow Abnormality

Erythropoietic Disorder

Hemophilia

Leukomas

Myelofibrosis

Thrombocytopenia

Chapter 14. Thesaurus Relating Blood Vessel Disorders

a) *Coagulation and Clotting*

    Embolus: Depends on occlusion.

        Arterial Embolism

        Cerebral Embolism

        Thromboembolism

    Thrombus: Aggregation of platelets and fibrin (also called Blood Clot).

        Fibrin

        Fibrinogen

        Platelets (also called thrombocytes)

    Thrombosis

        Arterial thrombosis

        Cerebral thrombosis

        Phlebothrombosis

        Thrombocytosis

        Thrombophlebitis

        Thromboembolism

    Aneurysm: Ballooning of a vessel at a weak spot due to blood pressure.

        Cerebral Aneurysm

        Dissecting Aneurysm

        Varicose Aneurysm or Varicosis

    Hemangioma

        Hemangiomablastoma

Hypovolemia

Infarction
        Cerebral Infarction ---------- causes stroke

        Myocardial Infarction ------ causes heart attack

Sclerosis
        Aoatic stenosis

        Arterial Sclerosis

        Atherosclerosis: An accumulation of fatty deposits.

Stenosis
        Pyloric Stenosis

        Vascular Stenosis

b) Inflammation

    Endocarditis

    Myocarditis

    Pericarditis

    Vasculitis
        Allergic Vasculitis

    Thromboangiitis

    Thromboendocarditis

    Thrombophlebitis

Chapter 15. Thesaurus Relating Dental and Oral Problems

Etymological Analysis

A: Prefixes

Group 1: Pain

Alge-, Algesi-

Group 2: Meaning of Dental
Dentin-, Dentino-, Dento-, Odont-, Odonto-

Group 3: Inside, Outside, Surrounding, Top

Apical- (Top), Endo- (Inward), Paro- (Surround), Peri- (Around), Perio (Around)

Group 4: Miscellaneous
Myo- (Muscle), Myxo- (Mucus), Ost- (Bone), Ortho- (Correct)

B. Suffixes

Group 1: Pain
-algesia, -algesic, -algia, -algic, -itis (inflammatory)

Group 2: Type of Development
-atrophy (poor nutrition), -blast (embryonic), -dysplasia (abnormal development) -genic (creating), -penia (deficiency)

Group 3: Dental
-odontia, -odontic

Group 4: Specialists (-ist, -on)
Endodontist, Periodontist, Orthodontist, Prosthodontist, Oral surgeon

Group 5: Surgical
-ectomy (extraction, removal), -tome (cutting tool), -tomic or -tomical (incision or sections of tissue)

Group 6: Disease or produced result
-ia (disease), -sis (result), -iasis (disease produced result)

Dental Problems	Thesaurus	Location	Own Notes
Coronary Decay	Apical Foramen	Enamel Crown	
Dentinitis	Caries	Dentin	
Gingivitus	Periodontitis	Gum	
Alveolitis	Odontobothritis	Alveolar Socket	
Periodontitis	Infection of Periodontium Eruptive Pocket	Cement periodontium	
Pulpitis	Pulp Inflammation	pulp	
Advanced Pain	Advanced decay	Root	

Dental Problem Classification

Types	Thesaurus or Examples	Own notes
Branch 1: Endodontist		
Pulp inflammation	Pulpitis	
Dental Caries	Dental Decay	
Branch 2: Periodontist		
Alveolar Osteitis	Infection of Tooth Socket	
Gingivitis	Alveolitis	
	Periodontitis Simplex	
Odontobothritis *(obsolete term)*	Eruptive Odontobothrion *(obsolete term)*	
Periodontitis	Infection of Periodontium	
Branch 3: Orthodontist		
Braces	Dental Braces	
Buck Teeth	Orthodontic Headgear	
Malocclusion	Correction of Malocclusion	
Branch 4: Prosthodontist		
Abutment	Supporting Implant	
Bridges	Cantilever Bridge	
Fixed Bridge	Cemented replacement teeth	
Crowns	Prosthodontia	
Denture	Removable Teeth	

COMPREHENSIVE MEDICAL THESAURUS

Dental Problem Classification

Branch 4: Prosthodontist (cont'd)		
Edentulous	Toothless	
Implants	Ni-Ti Implant	
	Implant Prosthesis	
Branch 5: Maxillofacial and Oral Problems		
Apthous Ulcer	Apthous Stomatitis	
	Canker Sore	
Bad Breath	Halitosis	
Bell's Palsy	Facial Paralysis	
Candidiasis	Oral Pruritus	
Cheilitis	Cheilosis	
Cleft Lip	Cheiloschisis	
Cranial Implants		
Labialis Herpes	Oral Herpes	
Maxillitis	Maxillary Inflammation	
Myositis	Muscle Inflammation	
Myxoblastoma	Malignant Mucus Gland	
Xerostomia	Dry Mouth	
Miscellaneous Terminology		
Abscess	Pus-filled hole	

Dental Problem Classification

<u>Miscellaneous Terminology</u> (cont'd)		
Apical Foramen	Coronary Opening	
Bruxism	Teeth Gnashing	
	Teeth Grinding	
Dental Calculus	Supragingival Calculus	
Dental Plaque	Sticking coating	
Dentinalgia	Dentinitis	
Dentinoblastoma	Malignant Dentinoblast	
Dentinoma	Odontoma	
Dentition	Odontotiasis	
	Teething	
Odontogenic	Odontogenic Fibroma	
	Odontogenic Fibrosarcoma	
Pulp Canal	Root Canal	
Glossitis	Tongue Inflammation	
Prophylaxis	Preventive Process	
Incisors	Front Teeth	
Molars	Wisdom Teeth	

Chapter 16. Thesaurus Relating Neck, Shoulder and Spinal Disorders

People, as they get older, tend to suffer from disorders in the shoulder and spine areas as well as others. Gradual deterioration of the joint structure or bone loss are due to Osteoporosis (   ). Some loss in height and weight and brittleness of the bones are quite normal. Such aging depends on individuals.

Osteoarthritis (   ) is caused by osteoporosis together with the loss of cartilage (   ) and fluid. These are acting as a cushion of the joint. The pain is caused by the growth of bony structure called osteophytes (   ). Osteoarthritis is also called "Degenerative Joint Disease" or "Osteoarthrosis." The pain usually starts in the morning. The stiffness pain may last for about 30 minutes of activity.

Rheumatoid Arthritis (   ) is a chronic systemic disease, which causes joint pain and limited mobility. Rheumatism tends to get worse and causes inflammation and growth of the joint lining called synovium (   ). It chemically destroys the cartilage, ligaments (   ), tendon (   ) and the bones. This disease is systemic, and therefore affects other body organs. Rheumatism starts even before senior age for some people.

1) *Osteomalacia Syndrome*

Osteomalacia is a deterioration of the bone structure. This causes pain in the lower spine, the shoulder and others.

Seniors tend to suffer from muscle weakness in the shoulder and thighs; and cramps. The syndrome involves bone pains and fractures of the hip, pelvis, ribs, and spine.

Malnutrition such as deficiencies in vitamin D and phosphorous are the start of problems. "Fat malabsorption causes vitamin deficiency because vitamin D is soluble in fat called Steatolysis."*

2) *Types of Shoulder Pain or Scapular Pain*

    a) Bursitis: Inflammation of the rotator cuff bursa .
        (Fibrous sac, containing fluid)
    b) Scapular Tendinitis or "Rotator Cuff Tendinitis".
        This is an inflammation of the tendon.

    c) Adhesive Capsulitis or Frozen Shoulder.

---

*Mark E. Williams, M.D. "Complete Guide to Aging & Health," Harmony Books, N.Y., 1995

d) Rotator Cuff Tears: Sometimes called "Pain of 50 years old."

Injuries of rotator cuff muscles and biceps tendon at the joint.

e) Osteoarthritis: The deformity starts usually at fingers. Joint pain of other body parts than the shoulder, such as the hips and knees, are also involved.

3) *Cervical Curve Area Disorders*
    a) Cervical Spondylosis (   )

    b) Cervical Vertebra Disorders: Compression in the neck.

4) *Thoracic Curve Area of the Spine*

    a) Spondylitis (   ): Inflammation of the spinal vertebra.

    b) Ankylosing Spondylitis (   ): This is also called Spondylosis (   ) meaning stiff spinal vertebra.

    c) Thoracic Hernia (   ) also called "Disc Hernia (   ) or "Vertebral Hernia."

    d) Spondylolisthesis (   ): Dislocated vertebra.

5) *Miscellaneous Spondylopathy (   ): Spinal Disorders.*

    a) Spinal caries (   ): Gradual spinal decay.

    b) Spondylocace (   ): Abnormal decay in the spine.

    c) Spondylosis (   ): Stiffness of a vertebral joint

6) *Lumbar Curve Area*

Lumbo- This prefix means "Lumbus" in Latin; "loin" or "waist" in English.

    a) Lumbago (   ): pain by a muscle strain.

    b) Lumbar Neuralgia or Sciatica (   )

    c) Lumbar Vertebrae (   )

7) *Sacral Area (   )*

a) Sacralgia (   )

b) Spondylolisthesis (   ): or "Spinal Cord Compression."

8) *Coccyx (   ) area*

    Coccygeal Pain (   )

9) *Spinal Deformation Disorders*

    a) Stooping (   )

    b) Osteocampsia (   )

10) *Rare Spinal Deformation Disorders*

    a) Spondyloptosis (   )

    b) Kyphosis (   )

    c) Scoliosis (   )

11) *Bone Marrow Disorders*

    a) Myelitis (   )

    b) Myelocystic Leukemia (   )

    c) Myelocystocele (   )

    d) Myelocystoma (   )

    e) Myeloma (   ): Marrow Swelling.

This is a special cancer of the bone marrow which causes pain and anemia.

    f) Myelomalacia (   )

    g) Myelopathic Anemia (   )

This is due to decreased production or red blood cell caused by malnutrition such as an iron deficiency in seniors' bone marrow.

Summary of Linguistic Analysis:

Prefixes	Examples	Meanings Prefixes
Cervico-	Cervicodynia	Neck
Lumbo-	Lumbodorsal Lumbosacral Lumbar Plexus	Loin, waist
Myelo-	Myeloblast Myeloblastoma Myelocyst	Marrow
Osteo-	Osteocarcinoma Osteodynia	bone
Scapulo-	Scapulohumeral	Shoulder

COMPREHENSIVE MEDICAL THESAURUS

Thesaurus Relating Neck, Shoulder and Spinal Disorders

Related Words	Thesaurus and Examples	Individual Notes
Arthritis	Osteoarthritis Osteoarthrosis Rheumatoid Arthritis Spondyloarthritis	
Back Pain	Ankylosing Spondylitis Spondylitis Spondylosis Thoracic Hernia	
Bone Marrow	Leukemia Myelocyte Myelocytic Leukemia Myelopathic Anemia	
Bursitis	Scapular Bursitis Rotator Cuff Bursitis	
Cervical pain	Cervical Spondylitis Cervical Spondylosis Cervicodynia Compressed Neck Neck Pain	
Hernia	Disc Hernia	

Related Words	Thesaurus and Examples	Individual Notes
Hernia (cont'd)	Dislocated Hernia	
	Thoracic Hernia	
Lumbago	Lumbar Neuralgia	
Myelatelia	Myelodysplasia	
Myelocele	Myelocystocele	
Myeloma	Myeloblastoma	
	Myelinoma	
	Myelocyst	
	Myelosarcoma	
Myelopragia	Myeloparalysis	
	Myeloplegia	
Myelopathy	Myelitis	
	Myelomalacia	
	Myelomeningocele	
	Myeloneutritis	
	Myelopathic Anemia	
	Myelosclerosis	
	Myelosis	
Osteoarthritis	Osteoarthropathy	
Osteo-	Osteocarcinoma	
	Osteoma	
	Osteomalacia	

Related Words	Thesaurus and Examples	Individual Notes
Rotator Cuff Tears	Biceps Tendon Injury	
	Rotator Cuff Muscle Tears	
Sacralgia	Spinal Cord Compression	
	Spondylolisthesis	
Scapulo-	Scapulohumeral Injury	
Sciatic Pain	Sciatic Neuralgia	
	Hip Pain	
	Lumbago	
Shoulder Pain	Adhesive Capsulitis	
	Frozen Shoulder	
	Rotator Cuff Tears	
	Scapular Pain	
Spinal Fusion	Spondylosyndesis	
Spondylopathy	Spinal Caries	
	Spondylocace	
	Spondylolysis	
	Spondylosis	
Stiff Neck	Stiff Spinal Vertebra	
Stooping	Kyphosis	
	Osteocampsia	

Related Words	Thesaurus and Examples	Individual Notes
Tendinitis	Rotator Cuff Tendinitis	
	Scapular Tendinitis	
Thoracic Pain	Ankylosing Spondylitis	
	Disc Hernia	
	Dislocated Vertebra	
	Thoracic Hernia	
	Spondylolisthesis	
	Spondylosis	

Chapter 17. Thesaurus Relating Major Skeletal System

Major Skeletal System	Thesaurus	Individual Notes
(1) Skull	Cranium and Skeleton	
(2) Mandible	Lower Jaw	
(3) Clavicle	Shoulder Girdle	
(4) Cervical Bone	Neck Bone	
(5) Scapula	Shoulder Blade	
(6) Humerus	Upper Arm	
(7) Sternum	Mid-Thorax	
(8) Ribs	Thoracic Skeleton (12 pairs)	
(9) Spine	Vertebral Column	
(10) Pelvis	Basin, Lower Trunk	
(11) Radius	Forearm Bone	
(12) Ulna	Elbow Bone (Forearm Bone)	
(13) Thoracic Vertebrae,	Central Spinal Column (12 segments)	
(14) Intervertebral Disc,	Lumber Spinal Column (5 segments)	
(15) Sacrum	Sacral, Dorsal, Pelvis (5 segments)	
(16) Coccyx	Coccygeal beaklike Bone	
(17) Femur	Thigh Bone	
(18) Patella	Knee Joint Bone	

Major Skeletal System	Thesaurus	Individual Notes
(19) Tibia	Medial Leg Bone, also called Thin Bone	
(20) Fibula	Smaller Lateral Leg Bone	
(21) Carpal Joint	Wrist Joint	
(22) Ankle	Talus, Tarsal	
(23) Calcaneus	Heel Bone	
(24) Hallux	Big Toe	

Chapter 18 Thesaurus Relating Cerebrovascular Disorders

A) Lynguistic Analysis

    Cerebrovascular accident or cerebrovascular disease, cerebral anoxia are commonly called stroke.

    Cerebro or cerebral came from Latin "cerebrum" meaning "brain".

    Vascular means blood circulation which also came from Latin word "vasculum".

    "Anoxia" means poor supply of oxygen, and cerebral anoxia causes local damange in the brain, namely "multi infarct".

    "Apoplexy" is an obsolete terminology of stroke. Apoplexia means stroke in Greek.

Pseudo-thesaurus:

    There is a similar term called "cephal" or "cephalo" which means "head", not "brain". This word came from Greek. Citing an example, "cephalgia" or "cephalalgia" meaning headache.

B) Classification of Stroke

Thesaurus	Notes
Ischemic stroke (Ischemic attack)	Lacking of blood supply into the brain
Hemorrhagic stroke	Bleeding causes brain damage
Transient ischemic attack (TIA)	Returns normal within 24 hours
Minor stroke	Minor disfunction, reversible, or partial reversible*

*causes Multi infarct dementia

C) <u>Motor Disorders</u>

   1) Loss of Balance

Thesaurus & Pseudo Thesaurus	**Notes**
Ataxia	Poor coordination of balance, gait, etc.
Dizziness, Faintness	Momentary loss of balance without stroke.
Vertigo	An illusion of spinning

   2) Opposite Side Disorder, against side of brain damage.

Thesaurus	**Notes**
Hemiparesis	Paralyzed partially (opposite side)
Hemiplegia	Specific paralysis opposite to the brain damage.
Hemianesthesia	No sensation locally
Hemianopsia	Blind opposite to brain damage

   3) Swallowing Difficulty

Thesaurus	**Notes**
Dysphasia	Motor disorder of the esophagus
Achalasia	Corkscrew esophagus, sphincter trouble

   4) Motor Apraxia   Inability to perform a task

D) Communication Disorders

Thesaurus	Notes
Anomia	Word retrieval difficulty
Aphasia (Expressive)	Expressive difficulty
Apraxia of speech	Verbal apraxia
Dysarthria	Articulation difficulty, slurred or unintelligible
Paraaphasia	Partial aphasia

E) Amnestic Apraxia (or Amnesia)

Inability to perform a task due to dementia (Multi infarct dementia)

Thesaurus	Notes
Amnesia	Loss of memory
Dementia (Vascular dementia)	Due to stroke, Loss of memory

F) Cognitive Disorders

Thesaurus	Notes
Agnosia	No knowledge (gnosis means knowledge in Greek)
Apraxia	Inability to comprehend
Dysmetria	Inability to measure (metron means measure in Greek)
Receptive Aphasia	No comprehension

G) Causes of Stroke

1) Blood vessel disorders

Thesaurus	**Notes**
Blood clot	Solidification of blood
Atherosclerosis	Narrowing of the channel
Carotid artery plaque	Narrowing of the channel
Cerebral thrombosis	Blood clot formation
Cerebral embolism	Blockage of artery to the brain
embolus (circulating object)	Plugging of blood stream
plague	patch of atherosclerosis

2) Hypertension

    Congenital or myocardial causes

3) Congenital uncontrollable risk

    Sickle cell disease

4) Miscellaneous risk factors

    Smoking, obesity, inactive life style

APPENDIX

1: **Classification of Physicians**

   a) Clinics: General and Emergency

Practitioner	Family practitioner
	General practitioner
Internist	Cardiologist
	Endocrinologist
	Nephrologist
Emergency	Emergency physician
	Radiologist
	Traumatologist

   b) Clinical Specialists

Allergy	Allergist
Arthritis	Rheumatologist
Cancer	Oncologist
Intestine	Gastroenterologist
	Proctologist
Lung	Pulmonologist
Obesity	Bariatrician
Pain Control	Anesthesiologist
Podiatry	Podiatrist, Chiropodist
Thoracic	Thoracic Surgeon

Urology	Urologist

c) Specialist by Age and Sex

Pediatrics	Neonatologist
	Pediatrician
	Pediatrist
Seniors	Geriatrician
	Gerontologist
Women	Gynecologist
O.B.	Obstetrician

d) Miscellaneous Specialists

Bone Marrow	Transplant Specialist
Chiropractic	Chiropractor
Craniotomy	Cranio Surgeon
Cosmetic	Plastic Surgeon
Cutaneous	Dermatologist
Lithotripsy	Lithotriptor
Nerve	Nerve Block Specialist
	Neurologist
	Neurosurgeon
Orthopedics	Orthopedist

e) Optometry and Dental Specialists

Optometry	Opthalmologist
Dental	Dentist (also see page 307)

	Prosthodontist
	Orthodontist
Oral Surgery	Endodontist
	Periodontist

f) Supporting Physician

Etiology	Etiologist
Hematology	Hematologist
Histology	Tissue Specialist
HIV	Immunology Specialist
Pathology	Pathologist
Bariatrics (Obesity Control)	Bariatrician
Embryology	Embryologist
Neonatology (Pediatrics)	Neonatologist (Pediatrician)
Physiatry	Physiatrist (Test physical function)
Naturopathy	Naturopath
Rehabilitation	Occupational Therapist
Emergency Treatment	Traumatologist
Proctology	Proctologist

Appendix 2. Classification of Medical Studies

a) Autopsy Pathology

b) Biology

c) Cardiology

Cytology

d) Dermatology

e) Ecology (various influences of environment)

    Endocrinology (Metabolism)

    Epidemiology

    Ethnology (Human behavior, social costoms)

    Etiology (study of cause of disease)

g) Gastroenterology

    Gerontology

    Gynecology

h) Hematology (Oncology)

    Histology

i) Immunology

m) Microbiology

n) Nephrology

    Neurology

o) Opthalmology

    Otolaryngology

    Otology

p) Pathology

    Pharmacology

    Physiology

    Proctology (Treatment of colon, rectum and anus)

    Pulmonology

Psychology

r) Radiology

Rheumatology

s) Serology (Laboratory study of serums)

u) Urology

Other Medical Studies

Diagnostic Engineering

Environmental Health Study

Genetic Engineering

Surgical Pathology

Implant Technology

Transplant Technology

Lithotripsy

Audiology

Appendix 3. Complex Thesaurus related to "Angioma" and Etymological Analysis

Related Words	Complex Thesaurus	Individual Notes
a) Angioma	angioma cavernosum	
	cavernous hemangioma	
	cavernoma	
	corpus cavernoma	
b) Lumphangioma	cavernous lymphangioma	
	lymphangioma cavernosum	
	angioma lymphaticum	
c) capillary hemangioma	hemangioma simplex	
	strawberry hemangioma	
	strawberry mark	

Etymological Analysis of the above:
a) Angioma means "blood vessel tumor." "Oma" is "tumor" in Greek.

    Cavernosum or cavernous is from Lation "caverna" meaning "hollow."

    Hema is "haima" in Greek meaning "blood."

    Cavernous hemangioma is a cystic hollow blood filled tumor.

    Cystic means a cell structure. "Cav" is also from Latin meaning "cavity"

    Corpus is "body" in Lation, similar to "soma."

b)   Lymphangioma or lymphaticum is a benign tumor on the skin, dilated lymph vessels.

C) Capillary is "hairlike" in Latin, meaning "small blood vessels."

This kind of tumor is also called "strawberry hemangioma" or "strawberry mark."

Note: Some examples of "Complex Thesaurus" which include both Latin and Greek are listed in Part I, Chapter 1, and Part II, Chapter 7 and Chapter 8.

Appendix 4. Examples of Similar Thesaurus and Pseudothesaurus

a) Hemoglobin (Hb) vs Immunoglobin (Ig)

    Similarity
        1. Both are found in the blood
        2. Small ball shape of protein molecules

    Difference
        Hemoglobin: Oxygen carrying protein in red blood cells also called "Oxyhemoglobin."

        Immunoglobulin: Antibodies produced by the immune system also called "Gamma globulin"
            "B-lymphocytes"
            "Humoral antibodies"

    Kinds of Hemoglobin: H_bA, H_bA_2, H_bC

    Kinds of Immunoglobin: I_gA, I_gD, I_gE, I_gG, I_gM

b) Hemoglobin vs. Myoglobin

    Similarity
        1. Red color globin (small ball)
        2. Protein-iron compound
        3. Storing oxygen

    Difference
        Hemoglobin: Found in red blood cells

        Myoglobin: Found in muscles also in the urine

    Kinds of Myoglobin: Myglobinuria

c) Infarct vs. Infarction

> Similarity
>> 1. Local interruption of the blood supply
>
> Difference
>> Infarct: This is caused by anoxia, and found in necrosis tissues, vessels or organs.
>>
>> Infarction: This is caused by a lack of blood circulation
>
> Kinds:
>> Infarct: Anemica infarct, calcarious infarct, embolic infarct, necrotic tissues
>>
>> Kinds of Infarction: Cerebral Infarction (stroke), Myocardial Infarction (Heart Attack), Embolism, Thrombosis, Vasconstriction

Etymological Analysis of the above examples:

> Globin, Globule, Globulin: (Globus: Small sphere in Lation)
>
> Hemo: (Haima: Blood in Greek)
>
> Immune: (Immunis: Free in Latin)
>
> Myo: (Mys: Muscle in Greek)

Appendix 5. Thesaurus related to Heart Attack and Stroke

> Supplement to Part III Chapter 14 & 18

A) Cardiac Crisis and Brain Damages

1. Coronary artery obstruction

> Myocardial infarction -------------- Heart Attack
>
> Insufficient pumping --------------- Congestive Heart Failure

2. Carotid artery obstruction

> Cerebral infarction ---------------- Occulusive Stroke

3. Cerebrovascular accident (CVA) ---------- Hemorrage Stroke

B) Congestive Heart Failure

   1. Cardiomyopathy

   2. Valve stenosis

      (Aortic, Mitral, Tricuspid, Pulmonary)

   3. Arrythmia

   4. Atrial Fibrillation (Flutter)

   5. CHF (Left mitral valve or ventricular failure)

      Insufficient blood flow to vital organs affects the lung, and the brain damage of one side.

C) Vessel Crisis

   1. Atherosclerosis (Aortic Stenosis, Varicosis)

      Atheroma

      Fat Emolus, Plague

      Blood Clot, Blood Coagulation

      Thrombus

   2. Infarction, Occulusion

   3. Aneurysm

      Cerebral Aneurysm

      Disecting Aneurysm

      Fusion Aneurysm

      Varicose Aneurysm

         (Varicosis, mostly for seniors)

INDEX
PART I

Section A

abasia 110
abdominal 27
abdominal centesis 23
abdominal hernia 128
abdominal
 membrane 98
abdomino centesis 42
abdominoscope 17
abduction 14
abductor 14
aberrant 27
aberration 27
ablate 27
ablepsia 7, 37
ablepsy 7
abnormality 27
abort 16
abortion 27, 116, 117, 125, 129
abreaction 42
abscess 103
absorptiometry 24
absorption 50
acetaminophen 29
achalasia 52, 86
Achilles tendon 121
achlorhydria 28
achylosis 28
achylia 28
acid reflex 61
acne 98
acoustic 64, 83
acromegaly 62
acromion 111
acronym 4
acrophobia 98
ACTH 47
actinotherapy 19
activator 105
acute mastitis 83
acyesis 28
ADD 28
addisonism 28
ademoa 11
adenectomy 21
adenitis 28

adenocarcinoma 28
adenocele 11, 28
adenofibroma 11
adenohypophysis 62
adenoid 11, 28
adenolipoma 11
adenolymphoma 11
adenomycosis 11
adenopharyngitis 12
adenosarcoma 11
adenovirus 129
ADH hormone 30
adipo 57
adipocele 57, 77
adipose 44, 57, 77, 90
adipose tumor 77
adipositas 44
adipositas 90
adrenal cortex 28
adrenal crisis 28
adrenal gland 62
adrenal hormone 28, 46
adrenal virilism 82
adrenalin 28
adrenocortical 28
adrenocorticotropic 46
adynamic 33
aerophagy 28
afferent 13, 54
agenesia 28
agenesis 28
agglutination 105
agglutinin 27
aging 110
agnosia 28
agnosis 28
agonal thrombus 122
agoraphobia 98
agrypnea 70
AIDS 46, 70, 76, 118
ailment 95
akathisia 28
alactasia 75
albumin 29
alcoholic cirrhosis 78
alcoholic psychosis 102
alexia 52
alexis 52

algesia 95
algogenesis 93
algolagnia 77, 83, 108
alimentation 29, 89
allergic 64, 110
allergic rhinitis 64
allergy 29, 105
allergy test 45
alleviate 106
allograpft 66
allurement 90
alopecia 35, 50, 64
alopecia areata 64
ALS 3
alteration 43
aluminoid 29
alveolar 78
alveolar air 35
alveolar sac 108
alveolia 34
alveolitis 12
Alzheimer's
 disease 28, 49, 84,
amebiasis 52
amebic dysentery 52
amenorrhea 84
amestic apraxia 110
amnesia 28, 29, 84
amniocentesis 23
amphiarthrosis 30
Amyo 3
Amyotrophical Lateral
 Schlerosis 3
amyotrophy 86
ana phase 83
anabolic 29
anabolic steroid 29
anabolite 29
anal atresia 29, 101
anal stenosis 29
anal stricture 29
analgesia 29, 30
analgesics 95
anapepsia 6, 52
anaphase 44
anaphrodisiac 93
anaphylactic shock 105
anaphylaxia 29, 64, 105

anasthetic 29
anastomosis 22, 29, 73
anatomize 50
androgen 29, 82
androgenic hormone 122
andromania 82
anemia 7, 29, 43
anergic stupor 87, 117
anesthesia 89, 95
anesthetic 87, 88
aneurysm 30, 35, 127, 128
angina 91, 117, 127
angina pectoris 91
angina pectoris relief 88
angiocardiogram 16
angiocatheter 18
angiography 15
angioma 128
angioplasty 25
angophrasia 115
anhedonia 84
ankle 30
ankle edema 30
anklebone 120
ankyle, ankyla 30
ankyloglossia 123
ankylosing 107
ankylosis 30, 107
annoyance 89
anocathartic 42
anodyne 30, 87
anomia 49, 84
anophresia 92
anopia 7, 37
anopsia 7,37
anorexia 100
anorma 27
anoscope 17
anosmia 96
anoxia 30
antalgic 30
anterior 13, 14, 59
anterior lobe 78
anthracosis 27
antiaging
 chromosome 120
anticoagulant 30, 50, 65
antidiuretic 30

antidote 31
antipropagation 129
antipsychotic 124
antisocial 102
antispasmin 30
antitoxin 31
antivenin 31
anxiety neurosis 110
aorta 31
aortic aneurysm 30
aortitis 31
aortoclasia 32
aortomalacia 32
aortopulmonary 32
aortostenosis 32
apex 31
aphasia 52, 73, 84, 100, 115, 129
apheresis 31, 106
aphonia 31
aphrasia 31
aphrodisia 31, 93
aphthous 70
aphthous stomatitis 10, 41, 70
aphthous ulcer 10, 41, 70
apical 31
aplasia 29
aplastic anemia 29, 30, 65, 72
apnea 52, 113
apneustic breathing 52
apocrine gland 55, 119
apoplectic stroke 34
apoplexy 34
apparent 104
appendectomy 21, 35
appendix 31, 35
approximate 104
apraxia 28
apraxia of speech 110
Aran-Duchenne Muscular Atrophy 3
areolar gland 62
armpit 31
aroma 31
arrest 34
arrhythmia 86
arrtery 31
arterial fibrillation 86
arterial pressure 32
arteriography 32
arteriola 32
arteriovenous angioma 32
arteriovenous fistula 29, 32
arteriovenous shunt 32
arteritis 32
artery 31, 32, 128
artery clogging 91
artery coarctation 91
artery forceps 32
artery graft 63
artery-vein fistula 26
arthrocele 32
arthrocentesis 32
arthrochondritis 32
arthrodynia 32
arthroscope 54
arthroscopy 17
articular cartilage 32
articulatio cubiti 32
articulatio genus 32
articulatio plana 33
articulation 98
artificial fertilization 23
artificial respiration 106
asbestosis 27, 99
ascites 27
ascorbic acid disorder 109
asphyxia 44
aspiration 3
aspiration 38
assimilate 50
asthenia 33
asthma 33, 130
astragalus 120
astringent 118
ataxia 10
ataxic speech 100
atele 33
atelectasis 33, 44
ateleiosis 33
atelia 33
ateliotic dwarf 33
atelo 33
atelocardia 33
atelocephalous 33
atherectomy 18
athiaminosis 33
athlete's foot 122
atomizer 87
atonia constipation 33, 90
atonic impotence 33
atony 33
atopic 29, 33, 66, 110
atopic asthma 110
atresia 34, 44
atreto 44
atretometria 34, 44
atrial electrogram 16
atrichia 35
atrichosis 35
atrium 111
atrophy 3, 28, 34, 49, 59
atropic eczema 112
attack 34
attention deficit disorder 28, 76
attraction 80
auditory 64
auditory salpinx 108
auricle 53
auricula 53
auris 53
auriscope 53
auscultation 17, 34
auscultatory percussion 17
autonomic 91
autopsy 34
autopsy 87
autotroph 125
avulsion 34
awake 70
axillary 31, 34
axoneuron 88
azoospermia 34, 92

Section B

bacillary 100
bacillary dysentery 52, 111
bacillus 59, 99, 100, 114
back pain 109
backache 35
backward flow 107
bacteremia 46
bacteria 35, 59, 61
bacterial aneurysm 35
bacterial chromosome 128
bacterial pathogens 100
bacterium 46, 128
bag 35
balanced tension 123
bald 36
balloon angioplasty 25
balloon catheter 18
balneal 36
balneology 36
balneotherapy 36
bane 36, 100
baneful 36
Bartholin's duct 108
Bartholin's gland 46
basal layer 75
basal metabolism 59
basophilia 76
BCG vaccine 125
belch 28, 36, 47
belly 27, 128
bellybutton 126
benign cancer 40
beriberi 31, 74
berry aneurysm 30
beside 73
bile 36
biliary 36
biliary calculus 61, 78
biliary cirrhosis 36
biliary stone 61, 78
bilious 36
bilirubin 36
bilirubinuria 36
bipass surgery 25
bipolar depression 52
bipolar disorder 88, 102
birth 123
birth control 92
bisexual 71, 77
bladder 47
blastcyst 133
bleeding diathesis 50
blepsia 7
blepsy 7
blind gut 37
blind pouch 35
bloat 37
block 37, 91, 117
blood (haima) 65
blood clotting 65, 122
blood stroke 117
blood thinner 30, 65
blood vessel 126
bloodsucker 96
boil 37, 76, 119
bond 132
bondage 132
bone 94
bone atrophy 94
bone fractire 39
bone marrow 82, 114
booster dosage 51
botulism 35, 59, 100, 123
bowel incontinence 69
bowel resection 21
bowel twisting 129

bowleg 74
brachial 31
brain aneurysm 30
brain concussion 37
branchial fistura 23
breast 75
breast feeding 37, 75
breast pain 83
breath smell 64
breathing 38, 106
breech 37
brochiectasis 93
brochitis 130
bronchoscope 54
bronchoscopy 17
bruise 39
bubonic plague
bucca 39, 43
buccinator 43
bug 39
bulbocavernosus 46
bulbourethral 46
bulging 101
bulimia 39
buried sutura 23
bursa 35, 36, 119
bursitis 5, 32, 35, 36
buttocks 38, 39, 62
  102, 107
bypass 39

Section C

cachexia 34, 100
cachexy 34
cacochylia 6, 100
cacogastric 6, 52
cacophony 100
cacosmia 74, 97, 113
caked breast 40
calcaneous 120
calcemia 40
calcifenol 116
calcinosis 40
calcitonin 40
calcium calculus 40
calculus 40, 78, 126
calcus 27, 78, 108
caliectasis 40
calix 40 (or calyx)
callosity 40, 46, 74
callus 40, 46, 74, 78
calmant 40
calvous 40
calx 40

canal 40, 51
canalis 51
cancellous 40
cancer 40, 44
cancerous 41
candida fungus 11
candidiasis 10, 70, 122
candidosis 10
canker 41
canker sore 10
cantilever bridge 117
capsule 105
captivation 90
carcinectomy 21
carcinogen 41
carcinoma 41, 112
cardiac arrest 41, 64
cardiac catheter 54
cardiac cycle 104
cardiac edema 27, 119
cardiac murmur 86
cardiac pace maker 70
cardiac thrombosis 122
cardiac tonic 123
cardioverter 95
caries 41, 49, 99
carpal 41
carpus 41
cartilage 41, 46
cartilage graft 33
cartilaginous joint 73
castrate 41
CAT 15, 45
catabiosis 28
catalepsy 109
catamenia 84
cataplexy 42
cataract 110
catatonia 42
catatonic stupor 42
CAT-CAM 18
catharsis 42
cathartic 42
catheter 18
catheterization 18
caudad 14
cavernous 42
cavitas 42
cavity 42
cecal 42
cecitis 31, 37, 42
cecoptosis 42
cecosigmoidostomy 42
cecostigmoidoscopy 22
cecostomy 22, 42

cecotomy 20, 37, 42
cecum 31, 35, 37, 42, 125
celia 27
celiac block 37
celiocyesis 101
celioma 27, 125
celioncus 41, 125
celiorrhea 50
cell 105
cellular 42
cellular debris 103
cellulitis 42, 117
cenesthesia 96
centesis 42, 47, 70, 122
centripetal 70
centrocyte 70
centrum 70
cecotomy 125
cephalalgia 64
cerclage sutura 23
cerebellum 37
cerebral aneurysm 30
cerebral concussion 37,
  64
cerebral
  hemorrhage 34, 36, 117
cerebral infarction 34, 69,
  117
cerebral palsy 89, 95
cerebral vertigo 51
cerebro 37
cerebrosclerosis 37
cerebrovascular
  accident 117
cerebrum 37
cerumen 103, 130
cervical 87
cervical dilator 93
cervical fistura 23
cervix 87
cesarean 47
cessation 84
chalazion 118
chancre 43
chancroid 43
channel 40
channel ulcer 51
charlatan 104
charlatanic 104
cheek 39
chemical crystal
  arthritis 5
chest 116, 122
chest pain 127
chicken pox 113, 127

chief cell 133
childbearing 101
chlamydia 43
chlorosis 30, 72
chlorothiazide 51
choking 44, 91
cholangioma 44
cholangiopancreatogra-
  phy 16
chole 36
cholecyst 44
cholecystectomy 21
cholecystitis 44
cholecystostomy 22
cholelith 36, 61
cholelithiasis 116
cholelithotomy 78
cholesterol 44
chondral 41
chondritis 41
chondroarthritis 41
choriocarcinoma 99
chorion 99
chromatic aberrant 27
chronic hepatitis 66
chronic lung 48
chronic pain 95
chylous ascites 27
ciliary gland 62
circulation stasis 91
cirrhosis 66, 131
cirrhotic liver 65
clasia 107
cleansing 130
cleft 58, 107
cleptomania 78
clogging 91
clone 42, 85
cloning 42
closing 91
clostridium 59, 100
closure 34
clot 45, 122, 123
clot busters 122
clumping 91
coarctation 34, 91, 116
cognition 97
cognizable 97
coitus 71, 93, 111
coitus excitement 93
colectomy 21
colitis 70
colloid carcinoma 85
colon 54
colon stasis 33

colonic fistula 54
colonoscope 17, 54
color blind 45
colostomy 69
colp 45, 184
colpalgia 45
colpitis 45, 74
colpocele 45
colpocytis 45
colpodynia 45, 127
colpolypus 45
colpopathy 45, 127
colposcope 17
coma 45, 118, 126
comatose 45
comedo 45, 98
commensal 96
communicable 46, 54, 70
compulsion 45
compulsive 90
conceptus 45
condom 45
condyloma 45
confinement 104
congenital 66
congental spinal
   disorder 114
congestive heart
   failure 64
conjugate 61
conjugation 71
conjunctival test 45
conjunctive tissue 46
conjunctivitis 45
connector 132
constipation 90
constricting 91
constriction 34, 117
contagion 46
contagious 46, 70
contraction 115
convulsion 85, 97
convlusive 114
convulsive seizure 86
coprogogue 42
copulation 71
cor 64
cor dextrum 64
core 89
corium 112
corn 46
cornea 46
cornual pregnancy 46
coronary 64
coronary thrombosis 128

corpulence 90
corpulent 90
corpus vitreum 129
cortex 112, 130
corticotropin 47
cortisol 46
cortisone 46
costal 46
costotomy 20
Cowper's gland 46
craniotomy 20
crash 90
crazy 82
crepitation 47
crepitus 28, 47
crevice 58
CRF 47
cripple 47, 65
Crohn's disease 47, 69
crypt 47
crystal 116
crystalization 116
CT 15
cuboid 120
cuboidal tarsal bone 120
culdoscope 17
curdled milk 132
cutaneous 71, 112
cutaneous catheter 18
cuticle 71, 112
cuticular 112
cutis 112
cutis laxa 112
cutis marmorata 78, 112
cutitis 112
cycloplegia 89
cyesis 61, 101
cyetic 62
cyst 35, 47, 105
cystalgia 47
cystectomy 21, 35, 47, 116
cystic carcinoma 105
cystic duct 51
cystic duct stone 36
cystic fibroma 48, 105
cystic fibrosis 48
cystic neuroma 48
cystolith 36, 40, 128
cystoma 48
cystoscope 17, 54
cystostomy 22, 93
cyto 42
cytokine 42
cytokinesis 42
cytolithiasis 40

Section D

dacry 49
dacryadenitis 49
dead tissue 87
debilitation 57
debility 33, 57, 59, 130
decay 49
deception 64, 69
decompose 51
decomposition 49
decrement 49, 57
decrepit 28, 49
decrepitude 28
defective gene 48
defibrillator 25, 95
degenerate 49
deglutition 119
delirium 57, 96, 110
delivery 39, 49, 96
delusion 52, 64, 69, 92, 118
dementia 28, 49
demoralize 96
dental caries 49, 99
dental plaque 99
denture 49
depression 88
depressive psychosis 52
derma 112
dermal 112
dermatitis 113
dermatocyst 113
dermatology 112
dermatoma 113
dermatomyositis 5, 107
dermis 112
detention 104
deterioration 49
dextrocardia 14, 49
dextrocerebral 37
dextrum 14
diabetic 45
diagnostic 15, 16
dialysis 19, 49, 50, 53, 76, 80, 106
dialyzer 50
diaphragm 50, 98, 111
diaphragmatic hernia 50
diarrhea 50, 107
diathesis 50
dichotomy 50
dicumarol 50
didymitis 93, 121
didymus 93, 121

diencephalon 37
diffuse 97
digest 50
digital 50
digital angiography 50
digital fluoroscopy 15
digitalis 50
digitalis therapy 50
dilate 50, 56
dilated vein 127
dilated vessel 127
dilation 93
dilator 50, 56
diminish 49
diminution 106
diplegia 95
direct percussion 17
disappearance 106
discharge 53
discoid lupus
   erythematosus 79
diseased 85
disfigure 47
disinfect 97
disintegration 49
disk prolapse 109
diskinesia 33
disperse 50
dispersing agent 50
disruptive 124
dissect 47, 50, 51
disseminate 101
distad 13
distal 13
distend 50
distended vein 127
distention 50
diurectics 51
diuril 51
diverse 66
diverticular 35
diverticulitis 54
diverticulosis 54, 66, 107
diverticulum 35, 65, 196
division 108
dizziness 51, 128
DNA 121
DNA suction 25
dope 51
doppler 15
doppler imaging 51
dormant 51
dorsal 14, 35, 51
dorsal column 114
dorsal flexure 59

dorsalgia 35, 114
dorsiflexion 35
dorso 14, 51
dorsodynia 35, 52
dosage 51
Down's syndrome 49, 84
drain catheter 54
dream 92
drivel 51
drool 51, 111, 115
drowsiness 76
dry catarrh 131
dry cough 131
dry gangrene 87
duct 51
duct ectasia 40
duodenoscope 17
dwarfism 87
dysentery 52, 111
dysgraphia 76
dyslexia 52, 76
dyspepsia 6, 52, 54
dysphagia 52
dysphasis 31
dysphemia 115, 129
dysphonia 31, 52
dysphrasia 52
dyspnea 33, 52
dysthymia 52, 84
dystonia 42
dystrophy 3, 33, 34, 86

Section E

ear furuncle 103
earwax 103
eccrine gland 55
ECG 16
echocardiography 15, 51
E-coli 59
ectasia 50, 56
ectasis 50, 93
ectomy 47
ectopic pregnancy 46, 101
eczema herpeticum 66
edema 27, 119
EEG 16
efferent 13, 94
effusion 97
egg poisoning 59
ejaculation 53
eject 53
EKG 16
elastic cartilage 132
elbow joint 32

elective 129
electrocardiogram 15, 16
electrodynograph 16
electroencephalograph 16
electrograph 16
electrohemodynamics 16
elytrocele 53
elytrostenosis 53
emaciate 130
emaciation 100, 130
emasculate 41
emasculation 41
embolectomy 21
embolic 44
embolism 44, 65, 70, 122
embryo 53
embryoectomy 53
embryotroph 65, 125
emergency medical 96
emesis 53, 106, 129
emission 53
emotional 71
emphysema 119
empyema 103
encephalo 37
encephaloma 37
endaortitis 32, 53
endarterectomy 21
endarteritis 32, 53
endemic 95
endemic goiter 95
endemiology 95
endocardial 53
endocardianl 70
endocarditis 53
endocardium 53, 83
endoderm 70
endometrial 54
endometriosis 54
endometritis 54
endometrium 54
endoprosthesis 70
endoscope 17, 54, 70
endoscopic retrograde
 cholangiopancreato
 graphy 17
endotoxin 59, 100
endotracheal tube 54
enema 54
enervate 49
enervation 49, 106
engulf microorganism 82
enlarge 50
enterectomy 21
enteritis 47

enteroanastomosis 22
enterostomy 69
enterotoxemia 100
enterotoxin 100
entoderm 70
entreal 54
entritis 54
enzyme 120, 133
eosinophilia 76
epidermis 112
epilepsy 34, 85
epileptic stupor 87
epimysium 57
epinephrine 28, 54
epiphysis cerebri 98
episio 54
episiotomy 20, 54, 98, 102
epistaxis 88, 107
epithelium 57, 112
ergosterol 116
eroticism 77
erotomania 77
eructation 28, 36
erythema 55, 71
erythematosa 102
erythematous 55
erythrocite 65
erythrocytosis 99
erythroderma 55
erythropoiesis 65
erythropoietic 100
eschar 108
escharosis 108
eschartomy 108
Escherichia Coli 59, 100
esophagus 55
estrogen 55
etiology 55
etymology 121
eucrasia 55
euesthesia 55
eugenics 55
euphoria 55
euthanasia 55
euthenia 115
euthenics 55
evacuate 53
eviscerate 129
excision 106
excitation 55
exclusion 104
exclusion 106
excrement 55, 103
excrete 53, 55, 57
excretion 103

exdation 56
exhaust 49
exhaust 57
exhaustion 49
exocrine gland 48, 55
expansion 56
expectorant 103
expectorate 103
expel 106
external genitalia 102
extract 53
exudate 56, 103

Section F

face lift 57
facial nerve 88
faint 57, 126
fallopian tube 108
fantasy 69, 92
fascia 57
fasciectomy 57
fascinate 90
fasciotomy 20
fatal 51
fatigue 57
fatigure neurosis 88
fear-tension syndrome 98
febricity 58
febrile 58
febris 45, 58, 104
fecal 55
fecalith 33
feces 55, 57
fecundate 58
fecundity 58
feeble 57
feebleness 130
female homosexual 76
female urethra
 catherterization 18
feminine 57
feminist 57
femoral vein
 hemodialysis 26
fenestrate 47
fenestration 47
ferment 132, 133
fermentation 133
fertile 58
fertility 58
fertilization 92, 133
fetalis 58
fetoscope 17
fetus 45, 53, 58

fever 45
feverish 45
fiber-optic 17
fiberscope 18, 58
fibril 58
fibrillation 58, 86
fibrin 58
fibrinogen 58
fibroadenoma 125
fibrocystic pancreas 48
fibroid 125
fibroma 125
fibromyalgia 4, 5, 107
fibromyositis 5
fibrositis 4,5
fibrous band 121
fibrous sheath 57
field sobriety test 114
filament 58
fissurapudendum 58
fissure 37, 58, 107, 118
fissure pudendi 107
fissuyre 37, 107
fistula hemodialysis 19
fistulectomy 58
fistula 58
fixed phagocyte 82
flaccid 33, 95
flank 27, 29
flat wart 128
flatulence 28
flatus 28
flatworm 120
flesh 58, 108
flexible 59
flexion 59
flexure 59
flu 45
fluctuation 59
fluoroscopy 15
flutter 59
focal seizure 85
folds 75
Foley catheter 18
follicle 35, 42, 47, 59, 105
follicle stimulating 55
follicular cyst 105
folliculitis 37
folliculoma 59
folliculus 59
food poisoning 35
fracture 37
fragile 38
fragility 38
frail 38

frailty 59, 130
frambesia 132
freak 121
freckle 76
free phagocyte 82
frenzy 90
frontal lobe 78
fundus 37, 59
fundus uteri 59
fungal infection 59
fungal skin disease 122
fungate 59
fungicide 60
fungus 59
funic 60
funicular 60
funiculitis 114
funiculus 60, 114
furuncle 37, 76
furunclosis 37

Section G

galact 75
galactocele 61
galactorrhea 75
galactose 75
gall 36
gallbladder 35, 44, 78
gallstone 36, 61
gamete 61, 133
gametogenesis 133
gamo 61
gamogenesis 61
ganglion 61
gangrene 87
gasp 42
gastrectasia 56
gastric 61, 116
gastric hemorrhage 36
gastric lavage 76, 130
gastric ptosis 101
gastritis 116
gastro-acid 64
gastrocamera 18
gastroenteric 61
gastroenteritis 61
gastroesophageal
   reflux 66
gastrointestinal 61
gastroreflux 61
gastroscope 54, 70
gastrostomy 22, 61
gay 76, 82
gaze palsy 61

genemutation 43
generate 101
generic 93
genesis 44, 93
genetic engineering 44
genital herpes 111
genital reflex 61, 102, 111
genitalia 61, 102, 111
genitals 61
genitourinary 126
genu 74
genu varum 74
geriatrics 101
germ 61
German measles 83
gestation 25, 47, 62, 101
gibberish aphasia 73
giddiness 51
giddy 51
gigantism 62
gigantoblast 62
gingivitis 12, 49, 70
girdle sensation 133
glandula 62
glandular 62
glans 62
glans clitoris 62
glans penis 62
gliding joint 98
glioblastoma 8
globule 38
globulus 38
glossal 123
glossitis 123
glosso 123
glossodynia 123
glossology 121
glottidis 107
glottis 107
glucocoaticoid 46
glucogen 62
glucose 62, 75, 118
glucosuria 62
gluteal 62
gluteal tuberosity 38
gluteous 62
gluteral 38, 39
glycerin 62
glycerol 118
glyceryl alcohol 62
glyco 62
glycogen 62, 118
glycogenesis 46
glycosuria 62
goiter 95

gonads 121
gonorrhea 43
gouty arthritis 5, 62
graft 39, 63
granulocytic 43
gravid 62, 63
gravida 47
grease 130
green cancer 43
   (granulocytic
   sarcoma)
groin 63
growth hormone 62
gullet 55
gumboil 12, 70
gynecologist 90
gynecology 90

Section H

habitual abortion 116
halitosis 64
hallucinatory 96
hallucinosis 64
hamartoma 125
Hashimoto's disease 62
hay fever 64
heart attack 64, 69
heartbeat 95, 122
heartburn 61, 64
heat stroke 117
helper cell 65, 120
hemagglutination 65
hematemesis 36
hemato 65
hematology 65
hematoma 65
hematoplastic 65
hematopoiesis 65
hemicrania 91
hemiparaplegia 65
hemipararesis 65
hemiparesthesia 65
hemiplegia 65, 95, 96
hemodialysis 49
hemoglobin 131
hemolysin 65
hemolysis 65
hemolytic anemia 72
hemophilia 36
hemoptysis 36
hemorrhage 36, 107, 117
hemorrhoid 36
hemorrhoidectomy 21
hemostasis 65, 69

hemostatic 65
hemotroph 65
heotocholangitis 78
heparin 30, 65
hepatalgia 66
hepatic 78
hepatic coma 66
hepatic porphyria 101
hepatic vein 18
hepatitis 66, 78
hepatocirrhosis 66
hepatogastritis 78
hepto 78
hermaphroditism 71
hernia 107
herniotomy 20
herpes genitalis 113
herpes gestation 111
herpes sexualis 111
herpes
    simplex 11, 111, 113
herpes zoster 111, 113
heterodermic 131
heterogamy 92
heterograft 131
hiatus 66, 107
hives 67, 126
Hodgkin's disease 41
hoeplessness 52
homeotypic mitosis 85
homesick 89
homochromatosis 112
homolateral 72
homonym 4
homosexual 82
hordeolum 118
horn 74
horniness 74
horny layer 75
hydrocelectomy 21
hydrocortisol 46
hypersensitive 29, 105
hypertonia 123
hypertrophic 90
hypervolemia 92
hypnosis 76, 113
hypnotics 76
hypoacidity 28
hypochondriasis 88
hypoemia 7, 72
hypomensis 84
hypophysis 98
hypotension 94
hypovolemia 72
hypoxemia 30, 92

hyster 126
hysteralgia 126
hysterectomy 21
hysteric 82
hysterocyesis 126
hysterotomy 20
hysteroscope 18

Section I

iatrogenic 69
icterous 36, 73,
    131, 132. 69
ideopathic blood
    disorder 99
ilectomy 20
ileitis 70
ileostomy 22, 69
ileotomy 69
ileus 91
ileus infarction 44
iliac region 63
illusion 64, 69
imagination 69
immune 69
immunization 69
immunoabsorption
    dialysis 19
immunologic
    disorder 111
impact 97
impedigo 103
impediment 69, 91
implant 70
implantation 25
impulse 97
inactive 51
inborn reflex 105
incision 71
incontinence 69
incubation 51
indigestion 92
induced abortion 116
infarction 34, 44, 69, 70,
    117
infatuate 90
infected pharynx 117
infection 70
inferior 13, 36
inferiority complex 36
infiltrate 70, 97
inflamed nostril 106
inflammation
    9, 10, 11, 12, 70
influenza 70

infusion 70, 71
inguinal 63
inguinal hernia 63
inguinodynia 63
inherited disease 48
inhibit 117
inhibiting protein 69
inhibitor 117
injection 70, 71
inolith 116
insanity 88
insect 39
insecticide 39
insensibility 87
insidious 91
insomniac 70
instability 71
intestinal
    obstruction 129
instillation 71
insufflation 50, 56, 70, 71
integument 71, 112
integumentarysystem 112
intention 71
intention tremor 104
intracavitary radiation 19
intercostal 99
intercourse 71, 111
internal organ 117
interphase 83
interseptum 83, 84
intersexual 71
interstitial radiation 19
intertrigo 71
intervertebral 107
intestinal 54, 71
intestinal absorption 50
intestine 71
intracutaneously 70
intravenous 71
involuntary nervous
    system 129
iron deficiency 43, 112
ischemia 7, 30, 72
ischemic lumbago 72
isolation 104
itchy 72

Section J

jargon 73, 77
jargon aphsia 77
jargonize 73
jaundice 69, 131, 132
jaw 73

jaw bone 73
jock itch 122
joint 73, 115
jugular 73
jugulum 73
juice 118, 73
juicy 118
junctura 73
junctura synovialis 33
juvenile lentigo 76
juxta 73
juxtamural 73
juxtangina 73
juxtaposition 73
juxtaspinal 73

Section K

kakke disease 33,. 74
kakosmia 74, 97, 113
kera 46, 74
keratitis 46, 74
keratoiditis 74
keratoma 46, 74
keratosis 113
keratotomy 20
kernel 89
kidney 74, 87
kidney dialysis 26, 87
klaptomania 74
knee joint 32, 74
knock-knee 74
kyphoscoliosis 74, 109
kyphosis 35, 74, 109
kysthitis 74

Section L

labia 75
labia minora 89
lability 81
labio 75
labiodental 75
lacerate 47
laceration 47, 107
lacrimal 75
lactase 75
lactation 40, 75
lacteal 62, 75
lactin 75
lactose 75
laliatry
lalio 75
laliophobia 75
lalopathology 75

lalopathy 75
lamelia 75
laminar 75
laparoscope 18, 54
laparotomy 20, 2
laryngeal 122
laryngeal
    catherterization 18
laryngitis 122
larynogectomy 21
larynx 122
laser 19
laser angioplasty 25
latent 51, 91
lateral 13, 118
lateroabdominal 13
lateroflexion 13
lavage 42, 75, 76
laxative 42
layer 75, 117
lazy colon 33
leather bottle stomach 77
leech 96
leiodermia 113
leiomyoma 113
leiomyoma cutis 113
lemo 55
lemostenosis 55
lentigo 76
lentivirus 76
leprosy 65
lesbian 58, 76
lesion 113
lesion 76
lethal 51
lethargic 45, 76, 123
lethargy 45, 118, 123
leucocyte 75
leukemia 41
leukemia cutis 77
leukocythemia 77
leukocytoma 76
leukocytopenia 76
leukocytosis 76, 77
leukoderma 76
leukoma 76
leukomia 76
leukopathia 76
leukopenia 76
leukophoresis 76
leukoplakia 76
leukopoiesis 76
leukorrhea 76
leukosis 76
leukotomy 77, 78

leukotoxin 76
levocardia 14
libidinous 77
libido 31
libido 77
lienteric stool 55
ligament 115, 121
limit 105
lingo 77, 121
lingual 77, 123
lingual frenum 123
linguistics 121
lining 77
linitis 77
link 132
linning 83
lipa 57, 77
lipacidemia 57
lipemia 115
lipids 44, 77
lipo 44, 77
lipoatrophy 77
lipocele 57, 77
lipodystrophy 77
lipofibroma 115
lipoid 57, 115
lipoidura 57
lipoma 44, 57, 119
lipomatosis 77
lipomyoma 77
lipopenia 77
lipoprotein 44
lipoprotein 77
liposarcoma 77, 115
liposuction 24
lips 75, 115
lithiasis 78, 116
litho 40
lithocytomy 40
lithogenesis 78, 115
litholysis 116
lithotomy 20, 53, 78, 116
lithotripsy 20
lithotriptor 116
lithotrity 116
livedo 78, 112, 113
livedo reticularis 78, 113
liver 78
liver resection 21
lobe 78
lobectomy 21
lobectomy 78
lobotomy 77, 78
lobular 78
lochia 78, 79

lochiometritis 79
lochiorrhagia 79
loin 79
loop diuretics 51
loose skin 113
lordosis 109
Lou Gehrigh's disease 3
lower abdomen 36
LSD 90
lues 79, 119
lumbar 79, 130
lumbar nerves 130
lumen 52
lumina 52
lunacy 70
lung 79
lung cancer 79, 99
lupas pernio 79
lupus livedo 78
lupus vulgaris 79
lust 111
lustful 77
luteal 131
lutein 131
lutenizing hormone 55
luteoma 131, 132
lympcytotoxin 79
lymph 79
lymph node 2
lymphadenitis 28, 79
lymphadenopathy 79
lymphangitis 79
lymphatic 79
lymphcytopenia 79
lymphcytopenia 79
lymphcytotoxin 79
lymphocyte 79, 120
lymphocytosis 79
lymphoma 41
lysergic acid 80
lysin 80
lysis 80
lyso 80
lytic cocktail 29

Section M

macerate 81
machismo 81
macilent 81
macrocephalia 81
macrocephaly 81
macrocytosis 81
macrocyte 82
macrocytic 82

macroencephaly 81
macromolecule 82
macrophage 82, 207
maculation 76
magnetic resonance
    imaging 15
malabsorption 82
malignant 82
malignant cancer 40
malnutirition 49, 82, 100
malocclusion 49
malodorous 82
malpractice 82
mammary 37, 75
mammary gland 75
mammilla 38
mammitis 38
mamography 16
mandible 73
mandibular 73
mania 88, 90
maniac 82
manic depression 52
manic depressive 82
marijuana 51
marrow 114
maschism 83, 92
mast 38
mastadenitis 38
mastalgia 38, 83
mastalgic pain 83
mastatrophia 38
mastectomy 21, 38
mastitis 82
mastodynia 38
masturbation 83, 92, 93,
    111
mean arterial pressure 84
measles 83
meatus 83
medical 13
medium 85
medium lobe 78
medulla 114
megadose 51
meiosis 25, 83, 85
melancholia 83, 88
melanoma 113
membrana 75, 77, 83
membrane 75, 83, 77, 132
meningcele 114
meninges 83
meningitis 35, 83
menolipsis 84
menopause 84

menorrhagia 37, 84
menorrhea 84
menostasia 84
menoxenia 84
menses 37, 84, 94
menstrual 84
menstruation 37
mental capacity 84
mental deficiency 84
mental disorder 88, 102
mental displeasure 84
mental retardation 84
mentality 84
mercy killing 55
meso 85
mesaraic 85
mesen 85
mesencephalon 84
mesenterial 85
mesenteritis 85
mesial 85
mesoderm 85
metabolism 50
metabolize 51
metaphase 83, 85
metastasis 85, 84, 124
metastatic 84
methothelium 130
metra 126
metralgia 84, 126
metria 126
metritis 126
metrocarcinoma 84
metrocele 84
metrodynia 126
microbe 61
microlithiasis 78
microorganism 61
micturate 126
micturition 126
micturition reflex 128
midwife 90
migraine 64, 65, 95
migrate 124
migration 85
migratory pain 85, 124
mind 102
miscarry 117
missed abortion 117
mitosis 25
moderation 114
monozygosity 133
monster 121
morbus 85
morphine 51

motor seizure 110
motor-neuron disease 3
mottle 78
MRI 15
mucinoid 85, 86
mucinous 85
mucoid 85, 86
mucosa 85
mucoserous 85
mucous 85
mucous membrane 83, 85
mucoviscidosis 48
mucus 77
muliebral 58
muliebrity 58
multigravida 86
multipara 86
multiple gene 86
mural 130
mural thrombus 130
muscle contraction 123
muscular atrophy 3, 100
muscular dystrophy 86
muscular sarcoidosis 86
muscular tumor 86
musculoskeletal 86
musculus bucinator 86
mushroom poison 59
mutilate 47
mutilation 47
myalgia 86
myasthenia 33
mycobacteria 35, 46
mycobacteriosis 35, 46
mycotic aneurysm 35
mytosis 60
mycobacteriosis 60
myeloblast 82
myelocele 114
myelocyte 82
myelocytic leukemia 82
myeloma 41
myoatrophy 86
myocardial 65, 69
myoclonic 114
myoclonus 114
myofacial pain
    syndrom 5
myoma 86
myopathy 56
myotomy 20
myotonia 86
myotonic 86
myotonic myopathy 3
myotrophy 86

myxoadenoma 86
myxofibroma 48, 86
myxoid 86
myxoma 48
myxomatosis 48
myxomatous fibrosum 48

Section N

nanism 87
nanosomia 87
nanus 87
narcolepsy 42, 76, 113
narcosis 87
narcotic 51, 87
narrowing 91
nasalpolypectomy 21
nasolacrimal duct 120
nasopharyngeal 83
nausea 64
navel 92
nebulizer 106
necropsy 34
Neisseria 35
Neisseria meningitis 35
neoplasm 48, 119, 125
nephritis 87
nephralgia 87
nephrectomy 21
nephron 88
nephropathy 88
nerve block 88
nervous exhaustion 88
nervus facialis 88
nervus olfactorius 88
nervus opticus 88
netlike mottle 78
neuralgia 88
neuroglia 88
neurasthenia 88
neurology 88
neuron 88
neuronitis 88
neuropath 88
neuraploca 61
neuroglia 88
neurosis 88, 93
neurotic disorder 88
neutrophilia 76
nightmare 92, 113
nipple 96
nitroglycerin 88
nitrostat 88
NMR 16
noctambulism 113

nocturia 88
nocturnal 88
nocturnal
    emission 53, 88, 92
nocturnal fantasy 92
normal discharge 84
nosebleed 37, 88, 107
noso 89
nosocomial 89
nosocomial infection 89
nosology 89
nosophobia 89
nosopoietic 69
nostalgia 89
nostalgic 89
nostomania 89
notal 14, 35
notalgia 35
nourishment 89, 125
Novocain 89
noxious 89
nuclear division 25, 44
nuclear magnetic
    resonance 16
numbness 95, 96, 123
nutrient 89, 125
nutriment 89
nutrition 29
nutritive membrane 132
nyctal 88
nyctalopia 88
nycturia 88
nympha 75, 89
nymphitis 75, 89
nymphomania 75, 89
nymphotomy 89

Section O

obese 57
obesity 57, 90
obligate 90
observable 97
obsess 90
obsession 88, 90
obstetrics 90
obstruction 69
obturation 91
occipital 91
occipital lobe 78
occlusion 34, 91
occult 91
ocular 56, 91
odontalgia 91
odontitis 91

odors 92
oil gland 91
oil secreting skin 12
oily secretaion 112
olfaction 92
olfactory nerve 88
oligemia 92
oligogenesis 92
oligomenorrhea 84
oligopepsia 6, 92, 100
oligospermia 34, 92
oliguria 92
omodynia 92
omphal 126
omphalocele 92, 126
omphaloectomy 92
onanism 92, 93, 111
oncocyte 41
oncogene 41
oncogenesis 125
oncogenesis 93
oncology 41, 125
oncoma 41
oncosis 41
oncovirus 125
oneirodynia 92
oneirology 92
onychialgia 92
oogamy 58, 92
oogenesis 58
oophorectomy 9, 41
oophoritis 9, 92
oophorocystosis 9
oophoron 9, 92
oophorosalpingectomy 9
oosperm 92
oozing 56
opening 93
ophthalmitis 56, 93
opia 7
opiate 87
opium narcotic drug 87
opsia 7
opsy 7
opthalmia 56, 93
opthalmologist 93
optic 91
optometry 93
oral cancer 11
oral candidiasis
  10, 11, 122
oral herpes 70
oral thrush 11
orbital 56, 91
orchid 121

orchiectomy 121
orchiditis 121
orchis 93
orchitis 93
organogenesis 93
orgasm 93, 111, 110
orgasmic maturity 110
origin 93
orthodontia 49
orthodontic 93, 117
orthogenic 93
orthopedic 93
orthopedist 93
orthopnea 93
orthopsychiatry 93
orthoptic 93
orthostatic 94
osmidrosis 74, 113
osmosis 97
osmotic diuretics 51
ospheric 92
osphresis 92
osteoarthritis 32, 94
osteofibrosis 94
osteomalacia 32
osteonecrosis 94
osteophytes 74, 94
osteoporosis 94
osteosarcoma 48
ostium 93
ostomy 22, 69, 93
otis 53
otitis 53
oto 53
otoscope 53
ovarian 92
ovarian cyst 9, 35
ovarian explusion 94
ovariectomy 9
ovariocentesis 9
ovariocyesis 9
ovariostomy 9
ovariotomy 9
ovaritis 9, 93
ovary 35
overweight 90
ovulation 94

Section P

pacifier 124
pacify 124
pain killer 95
paint threshold 95
palate 107

palliation 95
palliative care 95
palliative treatment 87
palpitate 95, 122
palpitation 122
palsy 89, 95, 124
pancytopenia 7, 30, 72
pandemic 54
panic 96, 121
panting 52
pap smear test 96
papilla 96
papillitis 96
papilloma 96, 112
papulation 98
papule 96, 98
parodontitis 98
paralysis 89, 95, 96, 124
paralytic 124
paralytic abasia 110
paralyze 96
paramedic 96
paranoia 88, 96, 102, 109
paranoid 96
paranoid disorder 88
paraplegia 95, 96
parasitic
  microorganism 128
paresis 96
paresthesis 96
Parkinson's disease 28,
  124
Parkinson's tremor 97
parodentium 98
parodontitis 98
parosmia 97
parotid duct 108
parotidectomy 21
paroxymal dyspnea 33,34
paroxysmal 97, 114
parturition 49, 97
partus 49, 97
passage 83
passive tremor 97
pasteurize 69, 97
patella 74
patent 93
patent airway 93
pathogenesis 97
pathogenic 46
pathological yeast 132
pathology 85, 89, 97
pathosis 85
pavor 121
pavor nocturia 12

pavor nocturnus 113
pectoral 43
pectoralis 43
pelvis 103
penumo 79
peptic ulcer 61
perceived constipation 90
perceptible 97
percussion 17
perforate 97, 107
perforation 107
pericardiocentesis 23, 25
pericardiotomy 20
peridontium 98
perineal 54, 102
perinectomy 54
perineotomy 98, 102
perineum 54, 102
periodontal disease 98
periodontia 98
periodontitis 49, 98
periodontoclasia 98
periodontosis 98
perioneal laceration 107
periosteum 41, 98
peripheral 95
peritoneal dialysis 19, 26
peritoneum 27, 83, 98
peritonitis 27, 98
peritonsillar abscess 104
permeate 97
pernicious
  anemia 30, 34, 72
pertussis 98
pervade 97
pervasion 97, 108
pest 39
pesticide poisoning 99
pestiferous 39, 46, 54
PET 16
petit mal seizure 110
phagocyte 82
phalloidine poison 59
pharyngitis 12, 70
phlebo 127
phlebogram 16, 127
phlebotomy 20, 71, 127
phlegm 103
phobia 98
phonocardiogram 17
phrenic nerve 98
phrenitis 98
phrenodynia 98
phrenopathy 96, 98
physiology 97

pierce 97
pimple 96
pineal gland 98
pink eyes 45
pipette 52
pit 109
pituitary 98
pivot joint 98
placenta 99, 132
placentitis 99
placentoma 99
plague 61
plaque 99
plasma 99
plasmapheresis 99, 106
platelete 99
plegia 89
plethora 99
pleura 99
pleura lining 83
pleural 99
pleuralgia 99
pleurisy 99
pleurodynia 99
plexor 17
plug 45, 91
pneumatocele 79
pneumococcus 79
pneumoconiosis 99
pneumocystis 99
pneumocystosis 99
pneumonectomy 22, 99
pneumonia 79, 99, 117
pneumonic plaque 99
pneumonitis 99
pneumothorax 99
pock 109
pockmarks 109
podalgia 100
podarthritis 100
podema 100
podiatrist 43, 100
podiatry 100
podium 100
poison 89, 100
poisonous 89, 123
polio 95, 100
poliomyelitis 95
pollinosis 100
polycythemia 99
polymyalgia 107
polymyositis 5, 107
porphyria 100, 101
porphyria cutanea 123
portal cirrhosis 78

positron emission tomography 16
posterior lobe 78
pouch 35
posterior 13, 14
precocious 101
precocity 101
pregnancy 58, 101, 125
pregnancy luteoma 132
premature 101
presby 110
presbyatrics 101
presbycardia 110
presbycusis 101
presbyopia 101
prevent 117
preventive 101
preventive care 117
previta 99
processus 74
proct 101
proctalgia 101
proctectomy 22
proctitis 106
proctoscope 106
proctotomy 106
prodigy 121
produce 101
progesterone 55
prohibit 120
proliferate 101
propagate 101
prophylactic 45, 101
prophylaxis 101, 117
proptosis 101
prosodemic 70
prostalgia 101
prostatauxe 101
prostate 101, 130
prostatectomy 22
prostatic calculus 116
prostatic hyperplasia 101
prostatic hypertrophy 101
prostatomegaly 101
prosthesis 101
prosthetist 101
prosthodontia 101
prosthodontic 117
prosthodontics 49
prostrate 49
prostration 49, 130
protein 111
protein metabolism 29
proteinuria 29, 102

protocele 106
proximal 13
pruriginous 72
prurigo vulgaris 113
pruritus 10, 72
pruritus cutaneous 113
pseudo 104
pseudoarthritis 104
pseudocyesis 104
pseudofracture 104
pseudogout 62
pseudopodium 100
pseudotumor 56
psychiatry 102
psychic 102
psychic contagion 102
psychic infection 102
psychoanalyst 102
psychoneurosis 88, 102
psychopath 102
psychopathic personality 102
psychoplegic 96
psychosexual 102
psychosis 70, 88, 96, 102, 110
psychotic 70
ptyalin 115
ptyalis 111
ptyalism 111
ptyalorrhea 111
ptyalosis 111, 115
pubic 61, 102
pubic region 102
pubis 102
pudendum 102
pulmonary 79, 91, 99
pulmonary edema 99
pulmonary embolism 99, 122
pulpitis 12
pulsation 95
pulse 95, 102
pulsus paradoxus 102
punch 97
puncture 107
purpura 102
purpura fulminans 102
purpura paulosa 102
purpura urticans 102
purulent 103
purulent edema 27, 103
pururigo 72
pururitic 72
pururitus 72

pus 56, 103
pyelo 40, 103
pyelocystitis 40
pyelogram 103, 126
pyelonephritis 103
pyemesis 103
pyemia 103
pyesis 103
pygo 107
pygomelus 103
pygopagus 107
pyelogram 40
pyoderma 103
pyogenic 103
pyometritis 103
pyo-ovarium 103
pyopericarditis 103
pyopoietic 103
pyorrhea 103
pyosis 103
pyothorax 103
pyotorrhea 103
pyroric stenosis 116

Section Q

Q fever 58, 104
Q wave 104
QRS complex 104
quack 104
quack doctor 104
quackery 104
quarantine 104
quasi bend 104
quasi reflex 104
quaver 104
quavery 104
quick 104
quinsy 104
quiver 104, 124

Section R

rabies vaccine 80
radiation theraphy 32
ramus 105
ramus bronchalis 105
range 105
range of motion 105
reaction 105
receiver 105
receptacle 105
receptor 105
recidivation 106
recovery 105

recrudescent 106
rectal constipation 90
rectitis 106
rectocele 106
rectoscope 106
rectotomy 106
rectalgia 101
rectum 101
rectus 101
rectus muscle 101
recuperation 105
recurrence 106
reflex 105
reflex bladder 114
regurgitate 129
regurgitation 107, 129
rejuvenation 55
relapse 106
release 106
relief 105
relieve 106
rem 106
remedy 105
remission 105, 106
removal 106
renal 74, 106
renal calculus 74
resection 21
respiration 106
respirator 106
respiratory choking 91
resting tremor 97
restoration 105
restrain 114, 117
retinal 91
retinitis 91
retinosis 19
return of symptom 106
revert 106
rheumatica 5
rheumatism 107
rheumatoid 107
rheumatoid arthritis 5, 32
rhinal 106
rhinitis 106
rhinolalia 107
rhinopathy 106
rhinorrhagia 107
rhinorrhea 107
rima 58, 107
rima oris 107
rima glottis 58, 107
roseola 83
rotator cuff tears 32
rubella 83

rubeola 83
rumination 107
rupture 107

Section S

sac 35, 105
saccharin 62
saccharogen 62
saccular 35, 108
saccular aneurysm 35
saccule 35, 105, 108
sacculus 35, 108
saccus 36, 105, 108
sadism 108, 111
saggital 13
saliva 51, 55, 108, 113, 115
salivary duct 108
salivary gland 108
Salmonella 36, 46, 100
salmonellosis
    35, 46, 59, 100
salping 108
salpingectomy 108
salpingioma 9
salpingitis 9
salpingocyesis 9
salpingopexia 9
salpingostomy 9
salpingotomy 108
salpinx 108
sane 108
sanitize 50
sanity 108
sap 118
sappy 118
sarcoid 108
sarcoidosis 108
sarcoma 48, 108
sarcomatosis 108
sausage poison 59
scab 108
scanning 15, 16
scapula 108
scapulalgia 111
scapular 111
scapulohumeral 108
scarlatina 108
scarlet fever 108
schizocaria 108
schizocephalia 109
schizocyte 109
schizogenesis 109
schizoid 109
schizophasia 109

schizophrenia
    42, 109, 96, 102
schizotypal 109
sciatic nerve 109
sciatica 109
scirrhoid 109
scirrhoma 109
scirrhous 109
scirrhus 109
sclera 109
sclerectomy 109
scleritis 109
sclero 3
sclerocataracta 109
sclerocornea 109
scleroderma 109, 113
scleroma 109
sclerose 109
sclerosing solution 109
sclerosis 109, 125
sclerostenosis 109
sclerotherapy 109
sclerotitis 109
sclerotomy 109
scoliosis 109
scope 17, 105
scorbutus 109
scrobiculous 109
scrotal cancer 35
scrotum 35
scurvy 109
sebaceous 47, 55, 57, 91, 112
sebaceous crypt 55, 91, 119
sebaceous cyst 55
sebaceous gland 55, 91
sebacious gland 119
sebacious layer 57
sebum 112
seclusion 104
secrete 53
secreted fluid 53
secretion 53
sedate 124
sedative 30, 40, 87
sedative hypnotic 30
seed 110
seep 97
seizure
    34, 86, 97, 110, 114
semen 110
seminal fluid 110
seminal secretaion 46
seminal vesiculitis 110

seminal vesicle 110
senile 28, 110
senile purpura 102
senility 28
sensate 110, 111
sensation 110
sense of smell 92
senselessness 118
sensible 105
sensitive 104
sensitivity 110
sensory apraxia 110
septic arthritis 110
septic bursitis 110
septum 111
serologist 111
serology 111
serosa 111
serosanguinous 111
serositis 111
serosynovitis 111
serotonin 111
serous 111
serous fluid 111
serous membrane 111
serum 99, 111
serum albumin 111
sex change 124
sex chromosome 111
sexual abuse 108
sexual arousal 93
sexual dysfunction 111
sexual perversion
    83, 108, 111
sexual reflex 111
sexual transmitted
    disease 111
shake 104
shaking palsy 124
sheath 77
Shigella 52
Shiga's bacillus 52
shigellosis 52, 111
shingles 111, 113
shiver 104
shoulder ache 92
shoulder blade 108, 111
shudder 104
shunt 39
sialogogue 112
sialoma 112
sialorrhea 111, 112, 115
sialosis 112
siccant 51
siccative 51

siccus rhinitis 51
sidero 112
siderocyte 112
sideropenia 112
siderosis 112
sidetrack 39
sigmoidoscope 18
sinusitis 45
sitology 89, 112, 125
sitosterol 112
sitotherapy 112
Skene's gland 47
skin 71, 76
skin cancer 112
skin grafting 113
skin implant 113
slaver 113
sleep terror 92, 113
sleep walking 113
sluggish 123
sneezing 113
sobriety 114
sociopath 102
somatomic 47
somniferous 113
somnambulism 113
somnolent 113
soporific 113
sore 117
soundness 108
spasm 97, 114
spasmatic 114
spasmodermia 114
spasmodic 114
spasmogen 114
spasmophilia 114
spastic 114
spastic hemiplegia 65
SPECT 16
speech dysfunction 95
sperm 110
spermacrasia 34
spermatocyst 110
spina 115
spina bifida 114
spina bifida cystica 114
spina bifida occulta 114
spinal caries 115
spinal column 114, 115
spinal cord 114
spinal curvature 74, 109
spine 114
spinitis 114
spirogram 115
spirometer 115

spittle 115
splanchinocele 115
splanchnic 115
splanchnodynia 115
splint 58
split 109
split personality 86
splitter 37
spondyl 115
spondylitis 115
spondylo 114
spondylodynia 114
spondylosis 115
spongy structure 40
spore 115
sporoblast 115
sporocyst 115
sporogenesis 115
sporulation 115
sprain 115
sputum 55, 103
stammer 115
stapling 24
stasis 91
STD 111
steatitis 115
steato 57, 115
steatoma 57
steatorrhea 57
stench 113
steno 115
steno 46
stenocardia 116
stenocostal 46
stenoscope 17
stenosis 34, 44, 91, 116, 117
stenothorax 34
sterility 28, 34
sterilization 41, 116, 125
sterilize 97
sternocostal 116
sternum 116
sternutation 113
sternutatory 113
steroid 29, 46
stethomytis 116
stetho 43, 116
stethoscope 43, 116
stimulation 110
stink 113
stomach 116
stomach resection 22
stomach ulcer 61
stomachalgia 116

stool 55, 57
strains 117
strange 104
strangulation 117
stratum 117
stratum basale 117
stratum cornea 117
strep throat 117
streptococcal 117
stretcher 56
striated muscle 129
stricture 116, 117
strider 52
stridulent 52
strike 97
stroke 34, 69, 91, 117
stuffing 45
stun 119, 126
stunning 118
stupefaction 89, 95
stupor 118
stuttering 115
sty 118
styptic 118
subclavian
    hemodialysis 26
succulence 118
succus 73, 118
suck 118
suckle 118
sudation 118
sudor 118
sudoresis 118
sudoriferous 119
sudoriferous gland 55
sudorific 118
sudorrhea 118
suffocation 44, 91
sulcus 118
superior 13, 27
supination 118
supine 118
supine hypotension 119
supine position 119
suppress 117
suppressor 117
suppurative 103
suppurative otitis 103
sutura dentata 24
sutura limbosa 24
suturea serrata 24
swallow 119
Swan-Ganz catheter 19
sweat 118
sweat gland 119

sweat gland 55
swelling 37, 119
swollen 50
swoon 119, 126
symbiont 93
syncope 119, 126, 127
synovial 77, 119
synovial bursa 119
synovial fluid 119
synovial
    inflammation 119
synovial joint 33
synovial tendon 119
synovitis 5, 119
syphilis 119
syphilitic 119
systemic lupus 79

Section T

T Cell 120
tabes 120
tabes dorsalis 120
tabescent 120
taboo 120
tachpnea 52
taenia 120
taeniasis 120
tamoxifen 120
tangible 97
tapeworm 120
tarsal bone 120
tarsalgia 30
tarsus 30, 120
TB 125
tear duct 49, 120
telomere 120
temporal arteritis 32
tendinitis 5, 32
tendon 121
tendon reflex 121
tendon sprain 115
tendonplastic 121
tenodynia 121
tenonitis 121
tenotomy 121
teras 121
teratism 121
teratogenesis 121
teratogeny 121
teratoid 121
teratoma 121
teratosis 121
terror 121
testalgia 93

testectomy 93
testicle 93
testicular duct 121
testicular vein 121
testis 121
testitis 93
testosterone 29, 122
thanatology 34
therapeutic dialysis 12
thermography 15
thiazide diuretics 51
thigh 122
thighbone 122
thora 43
thoracic 43, 46
thoracic muscle 43
thoraco 43, 122
thoracoabdominal 43, 122
thoracocentesis 23, 122
thoracodynia 122
thoracotomy 20, 43
thorax 43, 122
threpology 89
thrichonosis 125
throat 122
throb 122
thrombocyte 99
thrombocytopenia 7, 30
thromboembolism 122
thrombolytics 122
thrombosis 44, 70, 122, 128
thrombus 44, 122, 130
throxine 122
thrush 122
thyroid stimulating hormone 62
thyroidectomy 62
thyroiditis 62
thyrotropic hormone 122
thyrotropin 62
tinea 53, 122
tinea capitis 53
tiresome 120
tocomania 123
toenail 123
tomography 15
tone 123
tonia 123
tonic 123
tonicity 123
tonsilitis 12
tonus 123
toothache 91
tophus 62

topical 123
toponarcosis 123
torpidity 123
torpor 123
toxicant 100, 123
toxicology 123
toxin 89, 100, 123, 124
toxocariasis 89
toxoid 123
toxolysin 123
trachalgia 124
trachea 124
tracheitis 124
tracheo 130
tracheomalacia 130
tracheostomy 22, 130
tracheotomy 20, 130
tranquilizer 124
transfection 124
transfer 124
transform 43
transfusion 124
transmission 85, 124
transplant 124
transposable 85
transpose 124
transposition 85, 124
transposon 124, 128
transsexual 124
transversal 13
transvestism 124
trauma 124
traumatic 91
tremble 124
tremor 124
trichogen 125
trichoid 125
trichologia 125
trichomania 125
tricoma 125
tricopathy 125
trochoid 99
trophology 125
trophtherapy 125
trophy 3
tubal abortion 125
tubal ligation 41, 116, 125
tubal pregnancy 125
tubectomy 116, 125
tuberculin 125
tuberculosis 79, 125
tuberosis 125
tuberosity 125
tuberous sclerosis 125
tumor 48, 125

typhlenteritis 42
typhlitis 31, 42
typhlosis 7
typhlolexia 125
typhlosis 7, 37
typhlostenosis 42
typhlostomy 42
typhlotomy 22, 125
typhoid 125
typhus 125
typhus vaccine 125

Section U

ultrasound scanning 15
umbilical cord 60, 132
umbilical duct 132
umbilical hernia 126
umbilicus 126
unconcious 126
unquis 126
ureter 126
ureterolith 126
urethra 126
urethral 126
urethrostomy 126
urinary 126
urinary calculus 126
urinary tract 126
urination 126
urine 126
urinoscopy 126
urocyst 35
urocystis 35
urogenital 126
uterine 126
uteritis 126
uterus 126

Section V

vaccine 101, 124
vacuole 38
vagina 45
vaginal 54, 76, 127
vaginal stenosis 116
vaginitis 45, 54, 74, 127
vagotomy 21
vallecula 118
vallecula cerebella 118
valley 118
varicella 113, 127
varicoectomy 127
varicose aneurysm 30, 128
varicose vein 127

varicosis 127
varicotomy 128
varix 127
vascular stenosis 116
vasculitis 127
vas-deferens 114, 127
vasectomy 22, 41, 114, 127
vasodepressor 127
vasodilation 88, 127
vasopressin 30
vasospasm 127
vasovagal attack 127
vasovagal syncope 127
vein 127
vena 127
vena cava 127
vena cava syndrome 127
venepuncture 23
venesection 23
venipuncture 127
venogram 16
venom 100, 124
venomous 100
venotomy 127
ventral 14, 27
ventricular electrogram 16
venular 127
venule 127
vermin 39
verminosis 39
vertebra 114
vertebral artery 114
vertebral joint 114
vesica 108
vesical calculus 36, 108
vesicle 35, 36, 108
vesicular 35
viosterol 116
viral infection 46
virile 82
virilism 82
virility 82
viron 129
virulent 82, 124
virus 46, 61, 100, 124, 129
virustatic 129
viscera 129
viscerate 129
visceral nervous system 129
viscus 129
vitamin 116
vocal cords 129

vocal folds 129
voluntary 129
volvulus 129
volvulus
 neonatorum 129
vomit 53, 106, 129
vulva 102
vulvar 102
vulvectomy 102
vulvitis 102
vulvovaginal 102
vulvovaginitis 102

Section W

waist 130
wall 130
warts 110, 130
wash 130
wax 130
weak 130
wheezing 33, 130
whiplash 130
white exudate 10, 11
white patches 76
white plaque 61

windpipe 130
womb 126
word salad 109
worsen 130

Section X

xanchromatic 131
xanchromia 131
xanthic 131
xanthine 131
xanthinuria 131
xanthochromia 131
xanthochromic 131
xanthoma 131
xanthomatosis 131
xanthopsia 131
xanthosis 131
xanthous 131
xanthous race 131
x-chromosome 131
xenogenesis 131
xenograft 131
xenoparasite 131
xenophobia
xenophonia 131

xeransia 131
xeransis 131
xero 51, 131
xerochilia 131
xeroderma 131
xerophthalmia 131
xeroradiography 131
xeroradiography 51, 131
xerostomia 131
xerostomia 51
x-ray 16

Section Y

yawn 132
yaws 132
yeast 132
yellow cartilage 132
yellow disease 132
yellow fever 132
yogurt 132
yoke 132
yolk 132

Section Z

zona 133

zone 133
zonesthesia 133
zonula 133
zonula ciliaris 133
zonule 133
zonulitis 133
zygogenesis 71, 133
zygosis 71, 133
zygosity 133
zygosperm 133
zygospore 133
zygote 133
zymocyte 133
zymogen 133
zymogene 133
zymogenesis 133
zymogenic 133
zymology 133
zymolysis 133
zymoma 133
zymophyte 133
zymosis 133
zymotic disease 133
zymogenic cell 133